This book would be an exciting addition for any headache sufferer or someone who lives with a headache sufferer. It covers a multitude of possible causes and gives innovative drug-free remedies. This book demonstrates Bob Phillips' compassion and determination to help those with a very potential debilitating condition.

—Robert K. Beck, MD
Private Practice, Board Certified
in Otolaryngology
[Specialty in Head and Neck Surgery]

The invisible pain of headaches has plagued mankind throughout medical history. Whether the pain is sharp, severe, blinding, dull, nagging, or prolonged, headaches disrupt the sufferer's lifestyle and affect his or her demeanor. Author Bob Phillips offers a very practical, structured approach to types, causes, and treatment of headaches for everyday use.

—Gilbert J. Kucera, MD
Private Practice, Board-Certified
Medical Review Officer
[Specialty in Testing, Evaluation, and
Effects of Drugs in the Human Body]

As a primary-care physician, I am impressed with the comprehensive approach Bob Phillips takes in addressing the numerous causes and drug-free strategies to headache relief. As a result of reading this book, I will broaden my approach to traditional headache treatment, seeking to better address the root causes. I look forward to implementing longer-lasting management strategies for my patients and less acute treatment with medications. This is a must-read for clinicians who treat headaches and for anyone who suffers from them.

—Ron Yee, MD
Chief Medical Officer
United Health Centers of
the San Joaquin Valley

I have recently had the opportunity to read *Headache Relief at Your Fingertips*, written by Bob Phillips. I would like to add my recommendation and endorsement to this book.

I have gone to many lectures through the years on taking care of headaches. In this book, there are more treatments for headaches than I have known in my studies. I do not think I have ever seen a more complete evaluation of headaches all in one book in my whole life. I think this book covers everything I have ever thought about headaches—and more.

I think this would be a good book for any person to own who has acute or chronic headaches, but especially for those with chronic and recurring headaches.

—Ronald D. Smith, MD
Private Practice, Family Medicine
Northwest Medical Group, Inc.
Fresno, California
Recipient of the Prestigious
California Doctor of the Year Award

# Headache RELIEF

## AT YOUR FINGERTIPS

**BOB PHILLIPS, PhD**



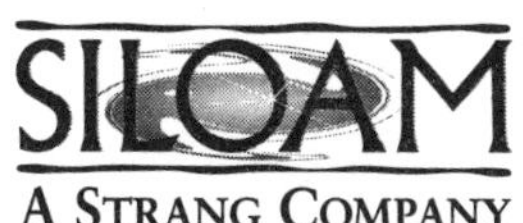


A STRANG COMPANY

Most Strang Communications/Charisma House/Siloam products are available at special quantity discounts for bulk purchase for sales promotions, premiums, fund-raising, and educational needs. For details, write Strang Communications/Charisma House/Siloam, 600 Rinehart Road, Lake Mary, Florida 32746, or telephone (407) 333-0600.

Headache Relief at Your Fingertips by Bob Phillips, PhD
Published by Siloam
A Strang Company
600 Rinehart Road
Lake Mary, Florida 32746
www.siloam.com



Cover design by Judith McKittrick
Interior design by Terry Clifton

Library of Congress Cataloging-in-Publication Data

Phillips, Bob, Ph.D.
Headache relief at your fingertips / Bob Phillips, Ph.D.
p. cm.
Includes bibliographical references.
ISBN 1-59185-636-1 (paper back)
1. Headache--Popular works. I. Title.
RC392.P48 2005
616.8'491--dc22
2004024805

AUTHOR'S NOTE: Names, places, and identifying details with regard to stories in this book have been changed to protect the privacy of individuals who may have had similar experiences. The people referenced consist of composites of a number of people with similar issues, and the names and circumstances have been changed to protect their confidentiality. Any similarity between the names and stories of individuals described in this book to individuals known to readers is purely coincidental.

This book is not intended to provide medical advice or to take the place of medical advice and treatment from your personal physician. Readers are advised to consult their own doctors or other qualified health professionals regarding the treatment of their medical problems. Neither the publisher nor the author takes any responsibility for any possible consequences from any treatment, action, or application of medicine, supplement, herb, or preparation to any person reading or following the information in this book. If readers are taking prescription medications, they should consult with their physicians and not take themselves off of medicines to start supplementation without the proper supervision of a physician.

05 06 07 08 09 — 987654321
Printed in the United States of America

# DEDICATION

I would like to dedicate this book to Dr. Robert Beck, Dr. Gilbert Kucera, Dr. Ron Smith, Dr. Peter Yao, and Dr. Ron Yee. Gentlemen, I appreciate your time, efforts, and suggestions in helping to make this book become a tool for headache sufferers.

# CONTENTS

*Lord, how my head aches! What a head have I! It beats as it would fall in twenty pieces.*

—William Shakespeare

# Introduction

Every now and then I have the opportunity to talk to groups about headache relief. Whenever I mention the subject, there is a great deal of interest. It was because of the interest generated and the suffering of many people that I decided to write this book.

My first exposure to the possibility of relieving headache pain within thirty seconds without medication came in the summer of 1980 while attending a psychological convention. At the convention, I was talking with Dr. Donald F. Tweedie Jr., an author and well-known Southern California psychologist. He mentioned that he was going to attend a pain and stress workshop that utilized acupressure. I said to him, "What is acupressure?"

Dr. Tweedie went on to explain that acupuncture is a stimulation of nerve endings by the insertion of needles into the body at certain points. Acupressure is the finger stimulation of these same points, only without the insertion of needles.

Since I already had a strong curiosity about acupuncture, I questioned him further. The thought of being able to help others with acupressure prompted me to enroll for the same pain and stress workshop.

Toward the middle of July I traveled from my home in Fresno to the Disneyland Hotel in Anaheim for the acupressure program. I must confess that I had no idea what I was getting into or how important it was to become in my life.

There at the workshop sponsored by the Center for Chinese Medicine, I met Dr. Tweedie, and we sat together. The gentleman who was leading the workshop was Ronald M. Lawrence, MD, PhD. Dr. Lawrence was the medical director of the Laurel Canyon Medical Clinic in North Hollywood. He had practiced Chinese medicine for eight years and neurology for more than twenty-five years. He was currently the West Coast director of the American Holistic Medical Association. He was also an assistant professor at the UCLA School of Medicine. In the past, he had been a research associate at the Rockefeller Institute of Medical Research.

Dr. Lawrence's interest in pain led him to become a founding member of the International Association for the Study of Pain. He was also a fellow of the American Academy of Angiology, American Geriatrics Society, American Academy of Family Practice, and the National Psychiatric Association. He was also board certified in psychiatry and electroencephalography. To say the least, I was impressed.

Dr. Lawrence gave us a brief history of acupuncture, which has been used by the Chinese for over five thousand years. He personally was trained in acupuncture in China, Taiwan, and Korea. He went on to explain and demonstrate how to help others with back and shoulder pains, facial pain, muscle cramps, stiff neck and shoulders, fatigue and tiredness, elimination of hiccups, insomnia, hypertension, abdominal pain, leg and hip pain, and the relief from headaches, including migraines and sinus.

The whole workshop was almost too much to absorb or even believe. As I drove back home, I was trying to think of how I would ever use all the information that Dr. Lawrence was talking about.

## DRUG-FREE HEADACHE RELIEF IN LESS THAN THIRTY SECONDS!

When I arrived home from the workshop, my wife was sitting at the kitchen counter painting on one of her art projects. After we kissed and said hello, I sat down beside her and proceeded to tell her about my time at the workshop.

As part of my sharing with her, I mentioned that Dr. Lawrence demonstrated how headaches could be eliminated in about thirty seconds without medication.

She smiled and said, "I don't believe it." She went on to tell me how she had been experiencing a splitting headache for over an hour.

I smiled and said, "Would you like to get rid of it?"

With a tone of disbelief in her voice she said, "Sure."

I took her hands and proceeded to massage them where Dr. Lawrence had shown us. I must say in all honesty that I too was a little doubtful if it would work. After about twenty seconds, she looked at me and said, "I hate to admit this, but it is gone." We both laughed.

That first encounter with acupressure massage encouraged me to continue to use what I had learned.

When I went to work the next day at our counseling center, our secretary, Doris, told me she had a severe headache. I asked her if she would like to get rid of it. She said yes, and I took her hands and began to massage the acupoints. All of a sudden she looked at me with great surprise and said, "It's gone." She asked me how I did that, and then I showed her how to do it on herself and others.

On another occasion, I was at my local bank talking with one of the bank's supervisors when an employee came up and said to the supervisor, "I need to go home. I have a terrible headache."

I looked at her and said, "Would you like to get rid of it?"

She was looking at me strangely. Who was this complete stranger in a bank offering to get rid of her headache? I did a quick explanation, and with hesitancy she offered her hands.

Within a few seconds, she looked at me and said, "What did you do? It's gone." As I walked away from the bank I thought to myself, *This is fun.*

In September of the same year, the Center for Chinese Medicine put on an acupressure workshop in Fresno, California. I decided to attend a second workshop to reinforce what I had learned in the first. This time the instructor was Dr. Pedro Chan.

Dr. Chan is a certified acupuncturist licensed by the State of California. He was practicing at the Acupuncture Holistic Center in Monterey Park. He comes from a Chinese medical family in Macao, where his father was a traditional Chinese doctor.

Dr. Chan served as a research associate at White Memorial Medical Center in Los Angeles. He is the author of five books on acupuncture. He was also the editor of *Acupuncture News,* a national professional monthly newsletter. In addition, Dr. Chan was the founder and executive director of the Center for Chinese Medicine. Dr. Chan has taught acupuncture to hundreds of doctors across the nation and lectured at various universities and medical centers.

From that day until now, I cannot tell you how many people I have helped obtain relief from headaches, hiccups, and other irritations. Frankly, it has been a great joy. Even my own children have helped their friends at school to get rid of their headaches.

## IS ACUPRESSURE FOR THE BELIEVER?

At various times I have been asked if acupressure is "Christian" or part of a cult of some kind. To me, asking if acupressure is Christian is like asking if eating apple pie is Christian. You have a choice. You can eat apple pie in moderation and thank God for it, or you can be a glutton when eating apple pie. Motivation is the key behind a great deal of things we face in life. Another example is money and how we use (or misuse) it. Do we use money to advance the kingdom of God, or do we bring discredit to His kingdom by what we purchase? The money is the same, but it is how we choose to distribute it that reveals the heart's intentions.

Just because someone pushes a nerve ending and releases endorphins does not make acupressure "Christian" or non-Christian. Some people have a tendency to "freak out" over anything they do not understand. I do not understand how a black and white cow eats green grass and produces white milk and yellow butter. Yet, I can enjoy the results.

So before you slam the book down, let me say one thing. Remember that long before the Chinese "discovered" these pressure points, God had already uniquely designed the body with the potential to mend itself. His Word says:

> For you created my inmost being;
> you knit me together in my mother's womb.
> I praise you because I am fearfully and
> wonderfully made;
> your works are wonderful,
> I know that full well.
>
> —PSALM 139:13–14, NIV

God created us and designed our bodies for healing. The question is, does God get the glory for His marvelous works, or does some person (or philosophy) claim the results?

I have been asked, "How does acupressure get rid of headaches?" Science does not have a complete answer, but we do know a few things. When you touch something hot, nerves send messages of pain to the brain along the nerve pathways. The brain then responds with the proper action to take, and the body responds accordingly.

When you massage certain acupoints, it sends some kind of stimulus message back through the nerve pathway to the central nervous system. The message proceeds up the central nervous system to the brain. The brain responds by sending messages back to the pituitary gland. The pituitary gland then releases endorphins. Endorphins are made up of enkephalins and complex lipoproteins, which are part of the endogenous opiate system. In plain English, endorphins are morphine-like, narcotic painkillers that the human body naturally produces. Endorphins reduce the pain that is felt in the body—including headaches.

Let me attempt to illustrate the concept for you. Have you ever had a stuffy nose? Most people have. I am sure you are no exception. Maybe you even have one right now as you are reading this book. If you would like to clear up your stuffy nose without medication, try the following exercise.

Place your two index fingers on your two front teeth (*the two top ones—the central incisors*). Next, slide both fingers to the two teeth on either side of your front teeth. (*These are the lateral incisors. Not too hard so far!*)

Next, slide both fingers to the two front (*top*) teeth that are very pointed. Can you feel the points? (*These are called your canines.*)

Those pointed teeth are also pointed on the tops of the same teeth. To find the top points, move both fingers up—to just under your two nostrils. (*Do you feel stupid yet?*) Move your fingers around until you find the top point of the two teeth. (*Trust me, they are there.*)

Find the very tip of the points of the teeth. Begin to press in and on the top of the points with about ten pounds pressure—fairly strong. Next, massage rapidly on the points while pressing down. (*You might want to close your door and draw the blinds. Some may think you have lost it.*)

Massage firmly and rapidly for about ten to fifteen seconds. If you have a stuffy nose on one or both sides—the massaging and pressure should open up the nasal passages, and you will breathe freely. It looks silly, but it beats nasal sprays.

Now, was that physical exercise—and the opening of your breathing passages—Christian or non-Christian? I think you get the point—literally. (Pretty scary stuff, right? I'll send you a bill.)

# PART I: BACKGROUND

CHAPTER 1

# The High Cost of Headaches

*There is no medicine like hope, no incentive so great, and no tonic so powerful as expectation of something better tomorrow.*[1]

—Orison Marden

"I don't know how much longer I can keep going! I've got to get some relief from these terrible headaches. I have two and sometimes three attacks a week. Sometimes I get so sick at work that I have to go home and go to bed. They seem to last for most of a day."

Mandy was thirty-five years of age and suffering from migraine headaches. She had been experiencing headaches since she was a teenager, and they were getting worse. Mandy would begin the day with a dull head pain in the morning. Soon she would become aware of a throbbing. It would be followed by a mild nausea that would tend to get worse. Sometimes the nausea would turn to vomiting and diarrhea. She would become dizzy and experience vertigo. Bright lights and noise added to her discomfort.

Her only relief was to get to a quiet place, turn out the lights, and lie down for several hours. During these times, the thought of food would make her feel sicker. Often during these periods of separation from people and activities, she would just cry over the excruciating pain and her feelings of aloneness.

This relentless pain began to affect her marital relationship. Her husband, Stan, would say, "We can never go anywhere or do anything, because you always have a headache." Mandy was hurt because of these comments. She didn't want the headaches. She didn't like being housebound by the pain. She felt guilty, hurt, and angry over something she could not control.

At work, Mandy felt that she was not holding up her end of the job. Her fellow employees were always filling in for her. Her boss seemed to be sympathetic, but she knew that he was getting a little irritated at her constantly leaving work sick. Every now and then she would hear comments from others that it might just be in her head, or that she was under too much stress. This only added to her guilt and confusion.

Mandy is not alone when it comes to her headache pain or how this dysfunction affects her social life. It is estimated 95 percent of people experience some type of headache pain in their life.[2] This would include mild to severe headaches.

Statistics indicate that one out of five women get them, followed by one out of twenty men. With migraine headaches, 61 percent last three and one-half hours, and 12 percent last longer than a day.[3]

It is estimated that more than $50 billion a year in lost productivity can be traced to headaches.[4] This represents somewhere between 92 million to 150 million lost days from work. Over half of these people miss two workdays a month and eight leisure days a year.

About $500 billion a year is spent on aspirin and other headache relief medications.[5] Headaches are big business for many of the pharmaceutical companies. It is estimated that individuals with severe headache pain attempt five different treatment options—over a period of three and one-half years—before they find relief. How much money have you spent on headache relief?

## HEADACHE HISTORY

Throughout human history, mankind has suffered from various physical complaints, illness, and disease. At the head of the list is probably the common cold. It is followed by headaches as a close second.

Primitive medicine attempted to deal with physical maladies through three basic hit-and-miss approaches. The first was to explore the possibility that there was some external cause for the complaint. Was the sickness passed on by a plague, dirty water, spoiled food, or some other source? The second was to examine the individual to see if there was some internal problem that was causing the illness. The third approach to the problem of headaches was the belief that they were caused by the influence of the stars, demons, magic, or as punishment from the gods.

Around 400 B.C. Hippocrates, considered the father of medicine, began to meticulously record observations of the diseases and injuries his patients experienced. He carefully noted their progress toward getting well and their failure to regain health. He began to develop an ethical code for physicians to follow, known today as the Hippocratic Oath.

In one of his writings, Hippocrates describes what sounds like a migraine headache:

> Most of the time he [the patient] seemed to see something shining before him like a light, usually in part of the right eye; at the end of a moment, a violent pain supervened in the right temple, in all the head and neck, where the head is attached to the spine...

Hippocrates, along with the Greek physician Galen (A.D. 131–201), believed that internal health problems—including headaches—were caused by the blood, phlegm, black bile, or yellow bile. It was believed that constipation caused a bilious liver to emit vapors that rose to the head and produced headaches.

Galen first introduced the term *hemikranion,* which means "pain on one side of the head." The same word in Latin became *hemicranium.* It was translated as *megrim* in the Old English. In French and modern English the word was translated as *migraine.*

A second-century physician named Aretaeus of Cappadocia (A.D. 30–90) describes what sounds like a typical migraine headache:

> And in certain cases the whole head is pained, and the pain is sometimes on the right, and sometimes on the left side, or the forehead, or the frontanelle; and such attacks shift their place during the same day.... This is called *Heterocrania,* an illness by no means mild.... It occasions unseemly and dreadful symptoms...nausea; vomiting of bilious matters; collapse of the patient...there is much torpor, heaviness of the head, anxiety; and life becomes a burden. For they flee the light; the darkness soothes their disease; nor can they bear readily to look upon or hear anything pleasant.... The patients are weary of life and wish to die.[6]

It was also believed that since blood (along with phlegm, black bile, and yellow bile) was the cause of many illnesses, the way to health was to drain "bad blood" from the patient. The process was called *bloodletting.* The draining of blood could be accomplished by the use of a knife or by applying leaches to suck out the blood. It is this process of bloodletting that sped up the death of President George Washington. In *World Book Encyclopedia* we read:

> Washington went for his daily horseback ride around Mount Vernon. The day was cold, with snow turning into rain and sleet. Washington returned after about five hours and sat down to

> dinner without changing his damp clothes. The next day he awoke with a sore throat. Between 2 and 3 a.m. on December 14, 1779, Washington awakened Martha. He had difficulty speaking and was quite ill. But he would not let her send for a doctor until dawn.
>
> James Craik, who had been his friend and doctor since he was a young man, hurried to Mount Vernon. By the time he arrived, Washington already had called an overseer and had about a cup of blood drained from his veins. Craik examined Washington and said the illness was "inflammatory quinsy." Craik bled Washington again. Present-day doctors believe the illness was streptococcal infection of the throat.
>
> Two more doctors arrived in the afternoon. Again Washington was bled. Late in the afternoon he could hardly speak, but told the doctors: "You had better not take any more trouble about me, but let me go off quietly. I cannot last long." About 10 p.m. on December 14, Washington whispered: "I am going. Have me decently buried, and do not let my body be put in the vault in less than two days after I am dead. Do you understand me?" His secretary answered: "Yes, sir." Washington said: "'Tis well." He felt for his own pulse. Then he died.[7]

Archaeologists have found skulls from as far back as 7000 B.C. with holes in them. These holes were cut with primitive stone knives in a process called *trepanning*. For headache sufferers, ancient mystics would bore a hole into the person's head to allow the imps, demons, or evil spirits to escape. The practice of trepanning for intractable headaches was used as late as 1630 A.D. by the British physician William Harvey.

Dioscorides was a Greek military surgeon who lived from A.D. 40 to A.D. 90. He believed that headaches could be cured by the use of electricity. He would apply *torpedo fish* (an electric ray) to the heads of those suffering with headaches. The shock from the fish would be enough to stun a man. Many of Dioscorides' health remedies remained in practice for fifteen hundred years.

The Chinese discovered and developed the practice of acupuncture about 2500 B.C. They used very sharp needles to stimulate nerve points in the body to relieve headaches and many other illnesses.

During the 1500s, a spinning chair was used for headaches and various mental illnesses. It was believed that if the individual was spun around and around, at a fast speed, it would force blood to the head. As the blood pressure would increase, it would help the people to throw up bad fluids in their stomach and force out their headaches or their mental problems.

In 2 Kings 4:18–20, there is the story about a boy who was in the field with his father when his head began to ache. This type of headache was most likely related to a fever. The event took place in the morning before the sun would become hot and cause sunstroke.

> And the child grew. Now it happened one day that he went out to his father, to the reapers. And he said to his father, "My head, my head!" So he said to a servant, "Carry him to his mother." When he had taken him and brought him to his mother, he sat on her knees till noon, and then died.

Through the centuries various headache remedies have been attempted. Some of the cures were mild like prayers and incantations, or the applying of herbs and oils rubbed on the head. It was believed that this would help drain excess negative fluids from the body. Other headache remedies were a little more strange:

- Drape reptile skins over the head and face.
- Wear the head of a dead vulture around the neck.
- Drink tonics concocted from cow manure to powdered flies and the testes of male beavers.
- Wear a boiled nest of a swallow around your neck for three days.
- A ninth-century British cure was to drink juice of elder seeds, cow's brain, goat dung, and vinegar.
- Peruvian Indians would cut a slit between the sufferer's eyebrows to provide an exit for the demons.
- Alaskan Indians and Polynesians would stomp on the person with a headache and wrestle with the person until the demons would become uncomfortable and want to leave.
- Mexicans would rub toads on the spot where the head would ache.
- Some would cover the headache sufferer with animal organs and feces, hoping to insult the demons so they would leave.
- Somewhere in the medical process, drugs like mandrake, belladonna, and opium were discovered to help alleviate headache pain.
- The early Sumerians discovered an interesting poppy plant—they called it the "Joy Plant."

# CHAPTER 2

# Theories About Headaches

*It is much more important to know what sort of a patient has a disease than what sort of disease a patient has.*[1]

—WILLIAM OSLER

From the beginning of recorded medical history, there has been a passion to discover a single cause for headaches, especially the migraine type of headaches. Everything from bad blood to dangerous foods and even to demons has all been blamed as the cause. Various physicians have collected data, made experiments, and have attempted to make application of their theories to the headache sufferer. In many cases this has led to misunderstanding, pain, and unreasonable conclusions.

Most physicians and scientists believe that headaches are a symptom of something else going on. You cannot have an event without a cause. They do not know why different headaches take on the form they do, nor do they know why headaches occur *when* they do. What they do know is that headaches are a process that produces a reaction that is experienced by the sufferer.

The bloodletting and demon theories have fallen by the wayside. However, that has not slowed reputable men of science and medicine in pursuit of the elusive cure for headaches. Let's take a look at some of these scientists and their theories.

Sicuteri believed that acute microcirculatory malfunctions are the main cause of headaches.

Du Bois-Reymond believed that headaches were the result of arterial spasms in the brain.

Mollendorff believed that headaches occurred because of loss of power in one side of the vasomotor nerves.

Liveing believed that headaches were the result of "nerve storms."

Horton, along with others, believed that *histamines, mecholyl,* and *reserpine* were responsible for headaches.

Kunkle believed that *acetylocholine,* which is present in the spinal fluid during attacks, was responsible for headaches.

Gibbs and Gibbs used the electroencephalograph (EEG) to discover electrical abnormalities during headaches.

Strauss and Selinsky used the EEG and discovered slow-wave abnormalities during headaches.

Whitehouse used the EEG to discover "positive spikes" in children with headaches.

Dexter noted that migraines that occurred during an individual's sleep happened during the REM cycle.

Dr. Harold Wolff, chairman of neurology at New York Hospital in the 1930s, did massive research on headaches. He has over 1,095 references to various studies. He noted an oxygen deficiency in a specific area of the brain during headaches. Dr. Wolff and many others began to study vascular influence as a causal factor. This led to studies on neurotransmitters and receptors in the nerve supply system. In recent years these studies have focused on a chemical known as serotonin or 5-hydroxytryptamine (5HT). *Serotonin* causes blood vessels to narrow. It also does not allow the body's natural painkillers, *endorphins,* to be released.

Dr. Zuzana Bic and Dr. L. Frances Bic believe that lipids and fatty acids, and the fat levels, in a person's body determine headaches. In their book *No More Headaches No More Migraines,* they suggest that nutrition is the key to controlling headaches.

Pete Egoscue, who is an anatomical physiologist, thinks that the alignment of the body is the key to headache relief. Egoscue states in his book *Pain Free—a Revolutionary Method for Stopping Chronic Pain,* "I have never known a migraine sufferer whose head, neck, and shoulders were not out of position in the characteristic mode of forward flexion."

Dr. Howard D. Kurland is a former professor of the Department of Psychiatry at Northwestern University Medical School, past president of the Association for General Hospital Psychiatry, former chief of psychiatric service of the Veterans Administration Research Hospital in Chicago, and senior attending neurologist at Evanston Hospital, Evanston, Illinois. He is also the author of *Quick Headache Relief Without Drugs.* Dr. Kurland believes that headaches are caused by three sources—vascular, sinus, and symptoms of serious disease. His entire book is devoted to relieving headaches through acupressure.

| THE OLDER VIEW OF HEADACHES |
|---|
| 1. Tension headaches |
| 2. Sinus headaches |
| 3. Migraine headaches |

Dr. John Mansfield, the author of *Migraine—the Drug Free Solution,* believes that migraine headaches are caused by food and chemical allergies.

Dr. David Buchholz, who served as director of the Neurological Clinic at Johns Hopkins and has published more than 150 scientific publications, believes that *all* headaches are migraines. They just vary in degree from very mild headaches, to tension headaches, to migraines, to the severe cluster headaches. He believes that what you put in your mouth will determine your headache potential. He states in his book *Heal Your Headache—the 1-2-3 Program for Taking Charge of Your Pain* that food and medications are the headache culprits.

| THE NEWER VIEW OF HEADACHES (ALL HEADACHES ARE MIGRAINES) |
|---|
| 1. Mild |
| 2. Moderate |
| 3. Severe |

Other physicians believe that headaches are influenced by:

- Female hormones
- Muscle tension
- Environmental factors
- Genetic heredity and family environment
- Psychological causes
- Low blood sugar levels
- Iron deficiency
- Accidents
- The headache personality
- Stress

It is abundantly clear that medical science does not completely understand or agree on the single source cause for headaches. Physicians and researchers have had significant success using various methods to bring headache relief to those suffering on a daily basis. Many headache relief medications on the market seem to help.

There is general agreement among those who study headaches (especially migraines) that they begin in childhood. They then tend to get progressively worse until around forty years of age. After forty, headaches seem to taper off for most people. Car sickness in children has been seen by many as a precursor to future migraine headaches.

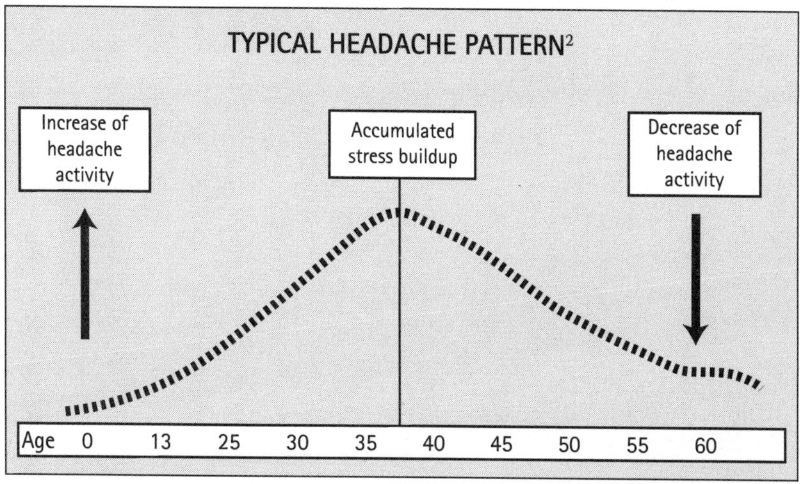


The question then arises, "What is the best method for me to pursue to find the headache relief I need?" This is the purpose for writing this book: to expose you to avenues that will best meet your need. But before we look at the various approaches to headache relief, we need to identify the various types of headache pain.

# CHAPTER 3

## Various Types of Headaches

*Headaches and pains are your body's way of telling you something. And have you ever noticed that your body becomes more and more talkative as you grow older?*

—Bob Phillips, PhD

Everyone has a DNA pattern that is completely unique to the individual. The same could be said of headaches. They are similar in nature, yet they are uniquely different for each person. Factors such as circumstances, pressures, environment, chemical imbalances, physical health, age, height, weight, diet, emotional stability, and personality all create a headache potential that is uniquely different for everyone, which makes it difficult to prescribe the same headache relief plan for everyone.

Having a headache is like a seagoing freighter ship with sand. You could fill the ship with sand until the water level became dangerously close to swamping the boat. Maybe it would only take another five pounds of sand to sink the ship. You decide that you won't add the extra five pounds, and you begin your journey across the ocean. The boat can carry this huge load of sand while traveling on smooth water. However, when the boat encounters an unexpected storm at sea, the waves easily pour over the edge of the boat, and it sinks. Why? Because there's not enough of the boat sticking out of the water to resist a surprise emergency. The boat's resistance level is too close to the level of the water.

A pressure headache is like the straw that broke the camel's back. A merchant had a camel that he used to transport his merchandise. One day he decided to haul some straw. He loaded his camel with a great burden of straw. He stepped back and looked at the load. He thought to himself, *I think my camel can carry some more.* With that, he loaded more and more straw on the camel. The burden on the camel grew to a tremendous size. Finally, the merchant said to himself, *I think I can add on one more piece of straw.* As he put the single piece of straw on top of the burden with the rest of the straw, the camel collapsed under the load. That piece of straw triggered the camel's breaking point. His tolerance level of stress was crossed, and his legs gave out. It was truly the straw that broke the camel's back.

The resistance level to stressors varies from person to person. Some people can carry a larger amount of stress burdens than others. But eventually, even the strongest person has a breaking or sinking point. Do you know what your breaking point is? How much of a load can you carry without sinking? Do you think it is important to know this information? If you don't want to collapse or sink physically, mentally, emotionally, or spiritually, this information is vital for your health and well-being.

Any number of factors can trigger a headache.

### A HEADACHE BY ANY OTHER NAME IS STILL A HEADACHE

Hippocrates, the father of medicine, believed that a physician should know about the nature of disease, drugs, and physiology, but his ultimate concern must be directed toward the individual. The physician cannot only treat the disease, but he must also treat the person.

| HEADACHE TRIGGERS | | |
|---|---|---|
| Sleep disturbances | Bright lights | Strong odors |
| Stress/trauma | Medications | Hormones |
| Weather | Depression | Dental problems |
| Motion sickness | Allergies | Hunger |
| Drugs/alcohol | Marital problems | Anger |
| Financial difficulties | Noise | Diet and food |
| Posture | Concussions | Caffeine |
| Work conflicts | Fear | Broken relationships |
| Anxiety | Eye disorders | |

This book on headache relief is not directed toward the physician, the scientist, or the pseudo-intellectual. It has been written for the layman who is suffering from headache pain and wants relief. Yes, of course, it is good to have a working knowledge about the science of human anatomy, but technical details as to how pain occurs along the nerve pathways is not the purpose of this book.

We will look at five major classifications of headaches along with sixty-three types, or causes, of headaches. Any one, or a combination, of these causes can bring about mild to severe headaches. Usually, there is more than one cause in the process. The increase of stressors can build up and spill over into a full-blown headache. The following classifications and types of headaches are those most people have experienced at some point in their life. The causes of headaches are listed in alphabetical order rather than the order of severity. See if you can identify with what follows.

## MAJOR CLASSIFICATIONS OF HEADACHES

Headaches have been mentioned in literature, studied by scientists, and treated by physicians for years. During the early 1960s, the National Institute of Neurological Diseases and Stroke invited a number of doctors to form a committee to discuss the classification of headaches. Their committee developed a list of fifteen major and fourteen minor headache classifications (types or causes). However, it was not until 1988 that the International Headache Society designed a more simplified classification guide for headache pain. It was a system to help standardize headache diagnosis, treatment, and research. Although many causes for headaches have been identified, the International Headache Society divided headaches into five major classifications: the *cluster* headache, the *migraine* headache, *mixed* headaches, the *sinus* headache, and the *tension* headache.[1]

*1. The cluster headache*

Sometimes Shane would just cry out with pain. He would hold his head and pace the floor wildly. He would attempt to rub his eye or one side of his head to get relief. He said that it felt like a nail had been driven in his eye and back into his brain on the right side. Shane was experiencing the walloping and knife-stabbing pain of a cluster headache.

Cluster headaches seem to strike men six times more than women. They are very strong during a man's twenties to forties. Cluster headaches can strike from four to eight times a day and recur for a three- to sixteen-week period. They come on quickly, and when the episode is finished, they disappear just as quickly. The attacks can last from fifteen minutes to several hours.

Cluster headaches are very painful. Some have likened them to a red-hot poker in the eye. Others say that they are like a drill boring into the head.

***The main signs of cluster headaches are:***

- Sudden and excruciating pain behind or around the eye on one side of the head
- Pain radiating to the temple, jaw, nose, teeth, and chin
- The affected area causing the eyelid to droop
- Eyes beginning to tear up and water
- Face becoming flush
- Nose may start congesting
- Sweating
- Pain when bending over or moving quickly

*2. The migraine headache*

Nancy is one of the many migraine sufferers who become physically incapacitated. Her excruciating pain will many times send her home from work. Over-the-counter painkilling medications don't seem to reduce her overpowering throbbing.

Often Nancy will become dizzy and lose her sense of balance. She will have severe abdominal pains, become nauseated, and vomit. Her headaches can last from as little as four hours and up to seventy-two hours.

Sixty-five percent of those with migraine headaches know another relative or family member that suffers with migraines. Migraines have been known to strike very young children. Migraines seem to increase in strength starting in the individual's twenties. They reach their height in the sufferer's mid-forties. Migraines are more common than diabetes or asthma. Migraine headaches are twenty times more common than cluster headaches.

Some migraines are known as *red migraines* because of a blush or flush in the face, similar to embarrassment or anger. Other migraines are known as *white migraines* because the face becomes pale and ashen. The individual looks drawn, haggard, and sunken.

Three questions can be asked to help determine a migraine headache from other types of headaches:

1. Have your headaches limited your daily activities (disrupted your work or daily routine) for one or more days in the last couple of months? ☐ Yes ☐ No

2. Do your headaches make you nauseated or sick, or do they cause you to vomit? ☐ Yes ☐ No

3. Does exposure to glare of light bother you a great deal when you have your headaches? ☐ Yes ☐ No

Migraines seem to follow four to five steps in their progression.

1. *Prodrome*—which occurs twenty-four hours preceding the migraine pain. During the *prodrome* there are subtle signs or disruptions that occur in about half of migraine sufferers. These signs can be in the form of nightmares, irritability, depression, euphoria, food cravings, excessive yawning, speech problems, and memory problems.

2. *Aura*—auras are visual impressions that are seen by the person with the migraine. Only about 15 percent of migraine sufferers experience auras. Migraines with auras are sometimes referred to as *classic migraines*. Migraines without auras are called *common migraines*. Auras usually precede the actual headache by about one hour. An aura can consist of flashing lights, brilliant colors, a shimmering, zigzag lines, blind or blank spots, or just spots. Colored spots that seem to move

around are called *phosphenes.* Sometimes you can experience phospenes without headaches when you apply pressure or rub your eyes.

3. *Headache—headaches* are intense and debilitating. The individual can become sick to the stomach, vomit, and ache all over. Muscles of the scalp become tender. Bright lights and noise intensify the pain. Movement adds to the discomfort. The person who experiences a migraine desires to lie down and rest in a cool, dark room.

4. *Resolution*—during the resolution phase the pain diminishes. It subsides with rest and sometimes sleep. Sometimes vomiting will end the headache. Intense emotional reactions like anger or fright can also end the headache.

5. *Postdrome*—in the *postdrome* phase, the pain stops. The individual feels tired, fatigued, and drained. They may feel mentally dull, and their muscles may ache. Eventually they return to feeling normal.

***The main signs of migraine headaches are:***

- General feeling of disorder
- Fever and chills
- Cold hands and feet
- Frequent urination
- Constipation or diarrhea in some
- Extreme sensitivity to light
- Sensitivity to noise
- Head seems to pound and throb
- Movement increases pain—especially bending over
- Dizziness, fuzzy headedness, and vertigo

- Ringing in the ears
- Numbness in the tongue and lips
- Head sore to touch
- Trouble concentrating
- Anxious irritability—restless and agitated
- Dejection, withdrawal, despair

While you were reading this chapter, a vast majority of Americans were experiencing a migraine headache. (If you stop reading at this point, it won't help them.) In a small percentage of cases in which a brain tumor is present, the symptoms experienced are similar to those experienced during a migraine headache episode. Therefore, it is recommended that you check with your family physician to rule out the possibility of a brain tumor as a possible cause of head pain.

*3. The mixed headache*

Mixed headaches are a "catch-all" category. When a headache takes on the combination of symptoms of the tension headache and the migraine at the same time, it is often called a "mixed headache." It can also refer to common daily headaches. Chapters four through seven list some of the headaches that come under the mixed headache category.

*4. The sinus headache*

Tiffany began to feel achy all over her body. She knew instinctively that her muscle pain and itching, irritated eyes were the first signs that a sinus headache was coming. She seemed to have more headaches when the cold and flu season was underway.

Every time her sinus cavities started to fill, she knew that she was in for head pain caused by the congestion. Tiffany was part of those 2 percent of the people who struggle with sinus headaches. She was also allergic to milk, wheat, eggs, and cat dander. This allergic reaction would sometimes help to bring on the itchiness in her eyes and the constriction of her airways.

***The main signs of sinus headaches are:***

- Inflammation and tissue-swelling of the mucous membrane inside the nasal passage
- Colored nasal discharge
- Drainage causing a sore throat
- Foul breath odor
- Dull aching in the frontal part of the head that can become quite intense
- General achy feeling in the muscles
- Itching and irritated eyes
- Sneezing
- Mood irritability
- Fatigue
- Fever and bacterial infection
- Blockage of the airways

### *5. The tension headache*

Gabriel seems to have recurring headaches that produce a dull throbbing. He feels as if there is a tight band around his head or as if his head is in a vice. His scalp even hurts. His headache is often accompanied by a great deal of muscle pain in his neck and back.

Gabriel has noticed that he is more susceptible to headaches when he is angry. Although his pain is annoying and uncomfortable, he is able to keep working despite the discomfort. He has what is commonly known as a tension headache.

Tension headaches make up an estimated 90 percent of all headaches that people encounter. Tension headaches are experienced three times more often by women than by men. Tension headaches are sometimes associated with depression.[2]

***The main signs of tension headaches are:***

- A dull throbbing and steady ache in the head—felt behind the eyes, on the side of the head, on the top of the head, or in the back of the head
- Head pain usually moderate rather than severe
- Excessive tightness, stiffness, and tenderness of muscles in the head, neck, and back
- A loss of appetite without nausea or vomiting
- Often pain on both sides of the head
- Often accompanied by fatigue
- Often accompanies emotional stress and strain
- Often accompanied by frowning and clenching of jaws
- Continuing to work or normal physical activity does not cause an increase of pain

This book is not meant to be a "fix-all" suggesting that you can eliminate headaches *forever* from your life. Don't you wish. There is nothing in science or the human experience that can make that kind of guarantee. This book is directed toward helping you recognize and manage the various stressors in your life that *trigger* headaches. By controlling these stressors, you can become more effective in raising your threshold level of resistance to headaches.

In the following chapters I will show you techniques on how to reduce the number of trigger causes, how to remain healthy, and how to get rid of *most* headaches in about thirty seconds to one minute without the use of medications and drugs. This will be worth the price of the book.

# PART II: CAUSES OF HEADACHES

CHAPTER 4

# Physical Causes of Headaches

*Those who do not feel pain seldom think that it is felt.*[1]

—SAMUEL JOHNSON

In the following pages we will examine the various sources of headaches. I have chosen to present these causes in the form of case studies so that you might readily identify with them. See if any of them might apply to your situation.

Physical causes of headaches come from three general sources. The first involves outside forces over which the individual may have no control. This could include things like accident-related injuries or unexpected motion. The second area includes inward bodily functions like fevers, tumors, and vascular disruptions. The last involves habits that include sleep patterns, exercise, and posture. As you read through the physical causes for headaches, become alert to any that may apply to you.

## UNEXPECTED CAUSES

### *Accident-related*

Correll was on his way to work on a busy Monday morning. As he entered the intersection at about thirty miles per hour, he was looking down at the radio to change stations. He did not see the speeding driver coming from his left run the red light.

The next thing he felt was the speeding car hitting his back left fender. Correll's car spun around and smashed into a parked vehicle. He was fortunate not to be killed or injured. He had only a few scratches. After talking with the police and having his car hauled off, he finally got to work about 10:30 a.m. He told his fellow workers the story and eventually settled down to work. It wasn't long before he began to feel a dull headache that began to throb to the beat of his heart.

Correll, like many people in accidents, tend to get headaches. Sometimes the headache is from a concussion, or it could simply come by bumping your head on the steering wheel. You may even experience headaches after tripping or falling over an object.

Just four days before writing this section of the book, I took my grandsons to the park. They asked me to join in a game of tag, and it was fun. At one point, I chased one of them up the slide. (Not the best thing to do.) I began to slip backwards, and as I attempted to reach down to grab the edge of the slide, my heels caught the opposite side, knocking my feet out from under me. I was now airborne about three feet off the ground. I landed on my back and knocked the wind out of myself. On top of that, it was a little embarrassing. When I got off the ground and caught my breath, I felt an instant massive headache. Hello. Of course, I would. I thought, *Well, at least I have a new illustration for my book.*

### *Motion-related*

Jeff had a difficult time with car sickness, especially traveling in the mountains. He would sit in the front seat or drive the car just to prevent becoming nauseated and having headaches. However, it did not stop with cars. He would get headaches on merry-go-rounds, roller coasters, and swings. Some of his worse headaches occurred as a result of traveling by airplane and experiencing "jet lag." I have come to believe that airplane seats were designed by someone out of the Inquisition.

## IN THE BODY

### *Brain tumor*

Linda was not a person to experience many headaches. So the explosive quickness of an excruciatingly painful, massive headache surprised her. She felt very weak and began to sense of loss of muscular control. Her vision was blurred, and her speech was slurred. She felt nauseated and soon began to vomit. Her husband talked with her, but she was disoriented. She was confused, and he could tell that she had some memory loss. He began to notice that Linda was having a mild seizure. Her husband knew that these were classic signs of something out of the normal. He was very wise and immediately took her to the doctor, who diagnosed her with a brain tumor.

### *Fever*

Elise had traveled to Africa as part of a Peace Corp mission. During her time in Nigeria, she came down with a sickness that produced a severe fever. The doctors at the hospital had to send for a special medication. During the two days it took for the medicine to arrive, the doctors used aspirin and cold baths to help keep her fever down. They had a difficult time controlling the headaches that accompanied her fever.

### *The vascular headache*

Rolanda tried to find the cause of her headaches. She didn't think that she was under any stress or pressure. Her relationships were all healthy, her diet was fairly normal, and she was exercising moderately. She could not think of any reason for the head pain.

Rolanda may be experiencing a vascular headache. A vascular headache can occur when there is an abnormal expansion of the blood vessels of the brain. This may take place within the protective covering of the brain called the *meninges.* It could take place in the blood vessels of the scalp. It may be caused by a fluctuation in the *serotonin* level. It might be the result of *temporal arteritis* (due to inflammation of the temporal artery), or it could be a sign of an *aneurysm.* An *aneurysm* is a ballooning of a blood vessel, which becomes a slow leak or a rupture and produces a hemorrhage in the head. If there are signs of mental confusion, loss of consciousness, or signs of a stroke, immediate medical attention is needed.

*Menstruation*

Sarah hated her "time of the month" with a passion. Not so much because of the blood flow, but because of the cramps and headaches that accompanied her change in hormone levels.

Women who are on their periods, those entering menopause, and those taking birth control pills can find themselves encountering headaches. This is due to their body adjusting to the variations in their estrogen level.

*Cough*

Cynthia had one of those infectious winter colds that had turned into a continual cough. The combination of sneezing, coughing, bending, and straining during her coughing bouts would often leave her with a mild headache.

*Disease*

Manny would have periodic headaches as a result of his diabetes. His struggle to balance the blood sugar levels of his body was not an easy one. Sometimes he would be high, and sometimes he would be low. As a result of this constant movement of blood sugar, he would often experience headaches.

Manny is not alone. People with diabetes, lupus, meningitis, and other diseases are often victims of headaches. I know of this on a personal basis in that my own daughter has been a brittle diabetic since she was three years of age. For over thirty years she has had to deal with this type of headache.

### *Dental causes*

Dental causes for headaches are a little more focused and easier to identify. This is because the source of the pain can be easily traced to a specific area in the body.

#### ***Abscess***

A few months before this writing, I went to the dentist with a broken tooth. He did some drilling, packed my tooth, and covered it with a temporary filling while a cap was being prepared. That evening my jaw and head began to experience whopping pain. I called him later in the evening and said, "I have to get some relief." He told me dig out the temporary filling, pull out the packing, and go to an all-night pharmacy for some antibiotics. I spent a terrible twenty-four hours with massive head pain all because of an infected tooth.

#### ***Bruxism***

Felix had a habit of grinding his teeth through the night. It was so loud that you could hear it in the next room. The grinding and gnashing of teeth is called *bruxism.* It occurs when a tense sleeper clenches his jaw, grinds his teeth, or clamps them tightly. This often causes a dull head pain behind the eyes and forehead and sometimes the cheek. Some people even grind or grit their teeth during the day. This is usually a sign of tension in the individual.

#### ***Chewing gum***

This is a no-brainer. If a person chews and chews all day long, this relentless grinding can tire the entire jaw area and lead to headaches. People who love to chew several packs of gum a day are not even aware that there is a relationship to their cud-chewing process and their head pain. Gum chewing can also be an indication of stress and tension. Often those who are under stress have the nervous habit to chew more rapidly as the stress level increases.

### *TMJ*

Several years ago, my daughter was involved in a car accident when a young man slammed into her car while at an intersection. She received severe whiplash, which led to neck pain and TMJ (temporomandibular joint) problems. TMJ is a disorder where the jaw becomes misaligned with the upper teeth.

It causes pain in the muscles where the jaw hinges. Chewing aggravates the tenderness in front of the ear. It hurts to bite down on anything hard like corn on the cob or apples. It is a dull, nagging pain, which proceeds to become a headache. The person with TMJ tends to cut his food into small bites so he does not have to open his mouth as wide. When he opens and closes his jaw, a popping or clicking sound can be heard. Chronic neck and back pain often accompany TMJ. Realignment can be accomplished with the help of a retaining device that is worn during the night and sometimes all day long.

### *Sexual*

There are a number of people who experience the bittersweet sexual headache. The pleasure of sex can be somewhat diminished because of the excitement, the energy expended, and the rise of blood pressure in certain individuals. During sex the blood pressure level can rise from 20–80 percent, thus bringing on a headache for those with hypertension problems.

Some interesting studies on Viagra and its relationship to headaches is being explored. Viagra dilates arteries in the entire body, not just the sexual organ. This expansion of blood vessels in the head can be a trigger for headaches in some men.[2]

### *Vision*

Cheryl had been experiencing headaches for several weeks. When she would read material, it was a little blurred. She found herself squinting a great deal and rubbing the muscles around the eyes. She eventually found out that she needed bifocal glasses. The optometrist also suggested that she change the level of her computer screen. He reminded her to take breaks more often and to add additional lighting in her office and at home, where she did most of her reading. Soon her headaches diminished.

Eyestrain, poor lighting, and the need for glasses should be one of the things you first look for when you have headache pain around the top of the eyes. The images sent to the retina may not be received properly. It is often wise to have your eyes checked for glaucoma or refraction errors when the focus is not clear.

## HABITS

*Poor breathing/air quality*

Stan had been cooped up in his small office all afternoon. He had his door closed so he could get an important project finished. At about 4:00 p.m. he began to notice the oncoming of a headache. The air was stale, and there was virtually no circulation in the room.

Often people do not realize that fresh air is vital to help ward off headaches. Sometimes we get so busy that we are not aware we are breathing with a very shallow intake of air. Deep breaths and fresh air can make a world of difference.

Air is filled with positive and negative ions. Some researchers suspect that an over supply of negative ions in the air accounts for many headaches. Remember how fresh the air smells just after a rainstorm? That is because the air is filled with positive ions.

Some people have a tendency to sleep with their heads under the covers. As a result, they do not breathe much fresh air. This can add to their potential of waking up with a headache.

*Disturbed sleep*

Eugenia was in her senior year at the university. She had taken a full load of eighteen units that semester. She was also working part time as a waitress in the evenings to help with school expenses. To make matters even worse, she was in the middle of her mid-term examinations. She had very little time to spend in getting adequate sleep. As a result, she had been fighting a headache for two days.

When I was directing our counseling center, one of the questions on our intake sheet was, "What is your sleep pattern like?" A change in sleep pattern, restless sleep, little sleep, or sleeping in an incorrect position can bring about headaches. A disturbed sleep pattern is also a strong indicator of depression.

*Exercise*

Hugo loved to work out at the local gym. He would lift heavy weights and would use the treadmill several times a week. He was not only attempting to build up muscle power, but he also wanted to develop his aerobic lung capacity by running.

Hugo was very disciplined and would push himself physically. All of his workouts were intense, and he would expend much effort. His body showed the results; he was as hard as a rock. He was happy about that. What he was not happy about were the headaches that would often accompany his extreme physical activity. His overexertion raised his blood pressure, and it resulted in much head pain.

*Neck disorder*

A number of years ago my wife's grandparents were sitting in their car at an intersection waiting for the light to turn green. All of a sudden a loaded cement truck struck them from behind. They were hurled into the intersection, and their car was destroyed. They were released within a short time with no major injuries.

However, the day was not over before they began to experience back and neck pain. For the next year her grandfather especially suffered with much neck pain and headaches from the whiplash of the accident.

Neck pain from pinched nerves can also cause headaches.

### *Poor posture*

Enrique had been suffering with headaches for several months. One day he mentioned his headaches to the physical therapist who worked out at the gym he attended. The therapist said, "Come with me. I want you to stand in front of the mirrors over at the corner of the building. In that way we can look at your body from various angles."

It didn't take long for the therapist to point out that Enrique's body was out of alignment. One shoulder was dipping lower than the other shoulder, which indicated that maybe his hips were out of alignment also. One shoulder lower than the other is typical of individuals under a great deal of stress. The therapist went on to point out that Enrique's head was forward about three inches instead of directly over the body. No wonder he was having headaches.

Enrique had developed the habit of sitting incorrectly in front of his computer at work. He walked with a funny gait and would stand with his feet and toes pointing outward instead of straight ahead. With a few well-chosen exercises, Enrique began to realign his body, and his headaches diminished.

### *Shopping*

How often have you left your list at home, or, after you arrive back home from the market, you realize that you forgot an important item? Sound familiar? For some, shopping is sheer joy. For others, shopping is literally a headache. The thought of driving in hectic traffic jams, finding a parking space, fighting through the crowds, looking for hours, walking a great distance, dealing with rude salespeople, returning damaged merchandise, and spending more money than you would like can be stressful. The next time you go shopping, make a conscience note of how much energy and time are expended.

*Sports*

Eric is a senior in high school, and he experiences frequent headaches after his involvement in sports. He plays with much excitement and expends a great deal of energy. But he can't figure out why he suffers the head pain.

What sports does Eric play? He plays football in the fall as a linebacker; he plays as a halfback on the city soccer team; he assists in teaching wrestling to the freshman class; and he is involved in karate whenever he has any free time. Hello, Eric. That may be the reason for your headaches.

*Weekend*

It took Sid awhile before he realized that there was a pattern to his headaches. They always seemed to occur on the weekends. On Saturdays and Sundays Sid did not get up as early in the morning. He did not have a schedule to keep. He did not have many pressures to face. His entire body reacted to the change in his schedule. Sid experimented with getting up the same time on the weekend as he did on the weekdays. When he began to keep his schedule more routine all week long, his headaches tapered off.

Some people have headaches on Sunday evening before the start of their working week. If this occurs on a consistent basis, it might be good to look at your work environment. Do you dread going to work on Monday? What is the cause? Do you have a conflict at work or an extra heavy workload? This will give you some clue as to the cause of headaches.

Physical causes when compounded by environmental influences can further increase a person's headaches. Let's look at the effect our environment has upon headache sufferers.

# CHAPTER 5

# Environmental Causes of Headaches

*No one else feels worse than the man who gets sick on his day off.*

—Bob Phillips, PhD

Many people are unaware of the strong effect that the environment has on triggering headaches. Toxic odors, smoke, and loud noises are very common headache producers. High altitude, glare, and heat can also influence the onset of headaches.

## ALLERGIES

One of the most subtle headache triggers comes in the form of allergies. Shauna really suffered from headaches in the springtime. She was extremely allergic to dust, pollen, and mold. Her sinuses would become inflamed and swollen. The combination of congestion and discharge wore her out. She was also allergic to cats. The cat dander would make her eyes swollen, her nose would run, and the headaches would come. Her sense of smell was highly alert to the smell of mold, especially in older homes.

## CHANGE OF WEATHER

When there would be a change in the weather, Kirk could feel it in his body. He had a built-in sense of any change in barometric pressure. The pressure change would often trigger headaches. Some of his hardest days were when the temperature dropped, the humidity rose, it was very cloudy, and the wind was blowing.

Many studies have looked at the effects of weather change and headaches. There is definitely a strong correlation, even though scientists do not understand why. This is another example of the conflict between the science of facts and the science of experience.

### DYNAMITE

Seymone had worked in construction most of his life. For the last ten years, his job was that of a "blaster." He would drill holes, set dynamite, and blow up granite. You would think that his headaches would come from the loud noise of the explosions. That may have helped, but it was not the main cause. The headaches he experienced came as a result of handling the dynamite with his hands and then wiping the sweat off of his forehead.

Many people do not realize that wiping grains of dynamite on your head can cause headaches. One of the major chemicals in dynamite is nitroglycerin. Nitroglycerin is a colorless and slightly oily liquid. It can be easily absorbed into the body through the pores, which is why doctors use it for heart problems. The nitroglycerin dilates blood vessels and helps to increase blood flow. However, one of the side effects of it is headaches.[1]

I personally learned this the hard way myself when I worked with dynamite as a young man. The men I worked with would not say a thing until after I rubbed my head and complained of headaches. They would smile and laugh. It was sort of an unspoken initiation rite to the world of construction workers.

### TRAFFIC COMMUTES

Bunnie lived in Los Angeles and had a two-hour commute each way from home to work and back again. She spent a minimum of twenty hours a week in freeway traffic. Often the smog was heavy and the traffic was slow. The combination of carbon monoxide, the tension of starting and stopping, the feelings of "road rage," and sheer boredom often produced painful headaches.

### GLARE

Travis couldn't bear being outside without his sunglasses. When he forgot them, he found himself squinting because of the glare. It hurt his eyes and brought about headaches.

Glare from sunlight, the bright light created by welding, and bright lights of oncoming cars at night cause headaches in many people. How do you feel when you are shopping in a store or working in an office where the fluorescent lights constantly flicker? Does it bother you? Have you ever looked at complicated visual images or visited an art gallery and felt the onset of a headache? The constant glare from computer screens is another instigator of headaches.

### HIGH ALTITUDES

My friend climbed Mount McKinley in Alaska a few years ago. The mountain rises to an altitude of 20,320 feet. One of his climbing partners got high altitude sickness. The pressure of the altitude made him sick and disoriented and brought on a headache. It became so bad that they had to help him off the mountain. He doesn't even remember being on the top of this high peak.

In recent years I have had the privilege of traveling to over thirty countries around the world holding seminars on ethics in leadership. One of those countries is Bolivia. When you travel to La Paz, Bolivia, you fly across Lake Titicaca and land at the airport at 13,600 feet above sea level. The Andes rise up around the valley to a height of 22,000 feet. You then drive from the airport down to La Paz, located at an elevation of 12,795 feet. It is one of the highest large cities in the world. At this altitude you can get headaches very easily. Most hotels provide lots of caffeinated tea to help with the headaches.

### LOUD NOISES

We live in a society where loud noise has become a way of life. We have bells on churches, sirens from emergency vehicles, and the constant drone of loud trucks. Booming sound systems blare from passing vehicles, radios and televisions are turned high, and yelling takes place at almost every sporting event. Are we surprised that there are headaches from the increase of noise?

### PAINT THINNER

I remember the first time I experienced what is called the "paint thinner" headache. I, along with another young man, was given the job to paint four rooms of a large building with shellac. It took about an hour for each room. We did not have any ventilation in the rooms.

By the time we got to the third room, we were laughing at almost anything and having the best time. Little did we know that we were becoming "high" on the fumes. When we finally finished painting and finally went outdoors for some fresh air, then we began to experience headaches.

### SMOKING

Devon worked in an office that was filled with smokers. She didn't smoke and hated it when she came home with her clothes smelling of cigarettes. After working in the office for about two weeks, she began to get headaches from the secondhand smoke. She knew she could not last long working for this company.

### SUNSTROKE

Domingo spent most of his days outdoors working as a carpenter. He had a constant battle with being overdressed or underdressed. If he wore too many clothes, he became overheated, and not wearing clothes that protected him from the sun left him vulnerable to its damaging rays. He found that when he began to lose body fluids and become dehydrated, he would get headaches.

## TOXIC ODORS

Researchers are finding an increase of headaches in people who are exposed to toxic chemicals and odors. Some cannot stand the smell of perfumes. Others who are exposed to pesticides and the fumes of pollution from factories experience head pain.

Welders who weld on galvanized metal experience zinc oxide headaches. The lead from paint, cosmetics, and gasoline bothers many people. Headaches can be caused from the fumes of formaldehyde used in plywood and insulation. Those living in mobile homes sometimes experience the formaldehyde headache.

# CHAPTER 6

## Emotional Causes of Headaches

*Half the spiritual difficulties that men and women suffer arise from a morbid state of health.*[1]

—Henry Ward Beecher

Emotions are very powerful influences in our lives. They can help to create great joy or be the cause of tremendous pain. Worries, anxieties, and concerns over health or finances can bring about massive headaches. Broken relationships, marital problems, and anger can generate much head pain. Stress from the job, trauma, and massive change also trigger headaches.

### ANGER

Travis had struggled with anger since his childhood. It started with small temper tantrums and fights with his brothers and sisters. It graduated to rebellion as a teenager and settled into yelling and angry outbursts as an adult. Travis did not see any relationship between his anger and his headaches until a day when one of his friends said, "Travis, when you don't get things your way, you simply blow your top."

Why do angry people blow their top? It is simply because people and situations do not work out as they would like them to. The person who "blows his top" can get angry with:

- His mate
- His children
- His relatives
- His friends
- His parents
- His fellow workers
- Injustice
- Himself
- Perceived danger
- Inanimate objects
- God
- Those in authority

### ANXIETY

Chavonne had felt like a failure most of her life. She had trouble making decisions. She struggled with a low self-image, and she worried about her health, relationships, and future. Chavonne continually found herself thinking about all the things that could go wrong in her life. Her constant thinking, worrying, and fear gave her anxiety headaches.

### BROKEN RELATIONSHIPS

Andrea had been deeply hurt a number of times in her life. It started when she was thirteen and her parents divorced. In high school, her best friend turned against her and passed on rumors about her. In college, her roommate stole her first real boyfriend.

After college, Andrea got a job in a bank. She worked hard for a promotion but was sabotaged by a fellow worker who was promoted over her. Just recently the man she was dating broke off their relationship. Andrea noticed that her headaches were coming more often and were more severe.

### CHANGE IN HABITS

Russell first heard it through the grapevine that his employer was going to have to cut back on the staff due to an economic downturn in the company. It wasn't long before he was called into his supervisor's office. He was told that those who had been with the company a long time were going to be given a severance package (the "golden handshake"). Russell was fifty-seven, and he was scared. He didn't have enough money for retirement, and he didn't know if anyone would hire him at his age. His skills were very limited. The change was overpowering, and so were his headaches.

We often resist change because of the fear of the unknown or the fear of failure. Change in habits, lifestyle, employment, or where we live causes disruption in our lives. Changes take time, energy, and often drain the emotions. We can become angry by being forced to change. We can become fearful because of the unknown future or loss of security. Change can become a trigger for mild to very painful headaches.

### CHILD REARING

Darla quit work to have her first baby. After the birth of her daughter, Jody, she soon became pregnant again. Within a year Darla had a set of twin boys. This was followed by a third boy a year and a half later.

Darla now had four toddlers.

Darla's parents lived three hours away and were not able to give her any relief when it came to babysitting. Her husband, Bill, was working long hours to earn enough to feed six people.

Darla felt tired, alone, and discouraged. She loved her children, but she also missed work and the satisfaction that accompanied it. She was now housebound to four demanding little ones. She longed for adult conversation, for some much-needed rest, and relief from the headaches she was experiencing.

### DEPRESSION

Jared had not felt good for several months. His normal energy level had dropped, and he was tired all the time. He just didn't seem to have the same motivation. He had an overwhelming sadness that he couldn't shake. There were times that he felt like crying, but the tears just wouldn't come.

He found that he was beginning to withdraw from his former activities, friends, and even from his wife. He began to feel that his family would be better without him. Jared began to think about ways he could die and still keep his life insurance policy intact. The dull cloud of depression was growing, along with his headaches.

Many people struggle with the giant of despair. That giant wants to throw them in the dungeon of doubting castle. Their depression takes away hope for the future and replaces it with hopelessness and headaches. You can be angry without being depressed, but you cannot be depressed without being angry. It is helpful for those who are depressed to consider whom they are angry with and/or what situation they are angry over.

### DILEMMAS

Adam was faced with a major decision in his life. It was a career move that could either make or break him. There were positive things about the decision, and there were negative things. For several weeks, he had been facing this decision, but he just couldn't seem to get off the fence. As his dilemma grew larger, so did his headaches.

Adam told a friend, "I don't want to make a final decision until I get all the facts." What Adam doesn't realize is that if he had all the facts, it would no longer be a decision. It would be a conclusion. Decisions are difficult because they are made without all the facts or guarantees.

### FINANCIAL CONCERNS

Kelli was not doing well emotionally. Most of her thinking involved her financial difficulties. It had been three years since her divorce, which almost forced her into bankruptcy. Her husband left her with two children and a stack of bills. He just disappeared and could not be found.

Kelli was working full time and would even do some part-time computer work in the evenings after the kids were in bed. She was worried because she was not able to save any money for medical or personal emergencies. She couldn't think about saving for her children's education or her future retirement. Kelli was living from paycheck to paycheck and from headache to headache.

### HEALTH ISSUES

Wally was under a load of concern about his wife's health. She had undergone chemotherapy for cervical cancer and was not doing very well. On top of her struggles, Wally just found out that his PSA levels for prostate dysfunction were extremely high.

Wally began to notice an increase in headaches that resulted from his concern about his wife's health and his own health. It was the first time in his life that he had to seriously think about the possibility of losing his wife and facing the prospects of his own mortality. These thoughts seemed to overpower his thinking.

### DISAPPOINTMENT (OR "LETDOWN")

Emerald had a terrific opportunity to show off her talents as a singer for an upcoming musical in her local community theater. She spent several weeks rehearsing the numbers. She would practice for three hours each evening. She knew that she would be facing strong competition, for others who would be trying out for the lead in the musical.

She was very nervous coming into the Saturday afternoon tryouts. Her nervousness grew as she sat there watching others perform. She knew it wouldn't be long before she would be up in front. All eyes would be on her, and the director of the musical would make his decision.

To her great joy and excitement, Emerald got the part as lead singer. She shared her good news with the family around the dinner table.

About 7:00 p.m., Emerald began to get a very strong "let-down" headache. These types of headaches come after a great deal of physical or emotional energy has been expended. Even though triumph is a wonderful feeling, it does cause quite a strain on one's physical body. The completion of an important task or the success from some event is often followed by the body shutting down for rest or relaxation. This abrupt change can trigger headaches.

### MARITAL PROBLEMS

Neil and Jennifer had been married for ten years. Everyone thought that they had a very happy and successful marriage. There were no outward signs of trouble. If you would go to their home, you would not pick up any negative vibrations.

Neil and Jennifer were very polite. They were not the type to yell and carry on. No, they were just the opposite. They were the silent type. They would hold in all their hurts, fears, and angers. They would hold in their dreams and ambitions about the future. They were silent about their resentments. They were silent about the fact that they had not been sexually active for one and one-half years. And they were silent about their headaches. "Not tonight, dear; I have a headache," was a reality for them.

### PERFECTIONIST

Juliana had grown up with a perfectionist father. He had demands for her that she had a difficult time living up to. When she got married and started to raise a family, she couldn't get away from the shadow of perfectionism.

Juliana's house had to be perfect all the time. The children's room had to be perfect even though they were small. Her husband was constantly hounded if he left anything out of place. Even when he would make the bed for her and put on all the decorator pillows, he couldn't do it right. Juliana would always make some minor adjustment to them.

Juliana could not relax. She had to be dressed perfectly. She had to cook to perfection. She had to be the perfect social host. She had to be the perfect community volunteer. Her car had to be clean and perfect. In fact, Juliana even had "perfect" headaches.

### POSTTRAUMATIC

Heather had a difficult time leaving the house. The only time she could go out was during the day—and only if someone was with her. Two months ago Heather was sitting in her parked car in the city parking lot, when a stranger carjacked her at gunpoint.

The man got in the passenger side and told her to drive to a secluded spot where he robbed her, raped her, and beat her up. It was a traumatic event in her life. Since that experience, Heather's anxiety, fears, and headaches had grown.

### WORK-RELATED

Jeremy had graduated from the university with a major in computer science. He soon got a job at a very progressive, high-tech company. It wasn't long before he found himself in a highly competitive, demanding, and stress-producing position.

His co-workers would backbite, undercut, and be generally unpleasant, making it a hostile work environment. Soon the conflict rose to such a height that Jeremy's stomach would turn at the thought of going to work. He developed headaches because of the work environment.

We often have to work with difficult people. It is usually the difficult people who eventually get fired from work, but not until they have destroyed the morale of their fellow workers. Kurt Einstein of *Success* magazine says that, "Eighty-seven percent of people who fail in work-related situations fail not because of *capability* but because of *personality*."

## SCHOOL

Kyle is ten years of age. He seems to be a normal and active boy except for one thing. He continually gets headaches that make it difficult for him to go to school. He missed quite a few days the last month.

It is not unusual for children to get headaches. However, when they become consistent and affect normal activity, it is important to see if there is a cause. Is there a pattern?

Kyle's parents did some investigative work. They talked to Kyle and his teachers, and they carefully questioned several of his friends. It wasn't long before they found the reason for Kyle's headaches. A bully had been picking on him. Not only had the bully pushed Kyle around and embarrassed him in front of his friends, but he was also demanding his lunch money, or he would beat him up. No wonder Kyle was having headaches.

## STRESS

Tonya's headaches were fairly predictable. She was a full-time mother of two small children. She had cooking, washing, diapers, and a husband to take care of. She was also taking four units at night school. Her husband would watch the kids while she went to school. Homework was done late at night and on weekends. She was actively involved at her church and occasionally participated in community activities. She had a hard time saying no to anyone who asked her to help.

Recently, Tonya's mother became sick and had to go to the hospital. She then took on the responsibility of visiting her mother and cooking meals for her father. She would even help her husband with the bookkeeping of his self-employed business. To all of this, she added the management of her headaches.

## TRAUMA

Trauma headaches are very similar to posttraumatic headaches. Both involve a crisis or trauma of some kind. The difference is that trauma headaches occur at the time of the trauma, not months later.

In the dictionary *trauma* is defined as "a wound, especially one produced by sudden physical injury." It is also defined in psychological terms as "an emotional shock that creates substantial (present—here and now) and lasting damage (future) to the psychological development of the individual."

I have included the trauma headache as sort of a "catchall" for any headache triggers that wound us physically or psychologically that are not in this list.

### VALUES CONFLICT

Tony comes from a family of strong religious faith. As a small child, he was taught from the Bible, and his parents stressed right from wrong. Positive moral character was lived out in the home by his parents. Tony did not come from what would be called a dysfunctional home.

Even though Tony strayed away from his parent's faith and became rebellious, he knew that it was a lifestyle that he didn't really believe in. At one point he even got in trouble with the law. Although his parents were disappointed in the direction of his life, they attempted to remain supportive. They didn't try to preach at him or lay guilt trips on him.

By the time Tony reached his twenties, he realized that the faith his parents had and the lifestyle they lived were something that deep in his heart he also wanted. It took a process of time for Tony to take his parents' faith and beliefs and make them personally his own. This inward struggle was the trigger for many of Tony's headaches.

This is a little-talked-about area. This type of headache comes from personal (individual) conflicts over values, morals, or issues of religious faith. It comes from not living up to the standards one has chosen or the ethics one deeply believes in.

I am not talking about imposed morals and ethics from others, but the guilt and failure to accomplish personal goals in the area of character and faith. The dichotomy of wanting to live a certain way and not doing it causes emotional stress. The person knows deep inside what is right to do, but he or she does just the opposite. For some, this is an area of deep concern. For others, they couldn't care less.

Values, morals, and ethics involve our conscience. Our conscience either accuses us or excuses us. A disturbed conscience creates anxiety and apprehension. The stress from this anxiety creates tension and then stress. This inner turmoil often leads to conflict and headaches. It has been suggested that there is no better tranquilizer than a clear conscience.

Yes, emotions can be very powerful causes of stress and pain, but we can exercise self-control over them. Likewise, we can exercise self-control over the kinds of foods we ingest that wreak havoc on our system.

CHAPTER 7

# Food Causes of Headaches

*The best doctors in the world are Doctor Diet, Doctor Quiet, and Doctor Merryman.*[1]

—JONATHAN SWIFT

It has been said, "You are what you eat." What you put *into* your body has a strong effect on what happens *on* your body. Many of the things we eat and drink can cause headaches. The difficulty is that we are either not aware of the cause-and-effect relationship, or we simply do not care.

## ASPARTAME

Sophia was very weight conscious. She had been on a strict diet for several months. During this time she noticed that she was having more and more headaches. She couldn't figure out why.

As part of her diet plan, Sophia would only drink diet sodas. Whenever she had any tea or coffee, she would only sweeten it with sugar substitutes. She attempted to be consistent throughout her diet.

What Sophia was not aware of was a chemical called *aspartame.* In many people aspartame is the cause of their migraines. In a survey done by the Centers for Disease Control and Prevention, it was found that the sugar substitutes like Equal and NutraSweet contain aspartame and cause headaches in a great number of users.[2] Some believe that aspartame is also a trigger factor in the decrease of serotonin levels that can help to lead to headaches. Aspartame is also found in many diet soda drinks. People who desire to have a diet drink that is caffeine free and aspartame free might consider Diet Rite Cola. If they would like to use a sugar substitute that is aspartame free, they might possibly use Splenda.

In one study involving seventy-five thousand women ages fifty to sixty-nine, it was found that they gained more weight using artificial sweeteners than those who did not use them. In another study it was found that diet soda drinkers ate more food and gained more weight than those who drank sodas with regular sugar sweeteners. Indications are that there is an increase of appetite after using aspartame. It is estimated that twenty pounds of aspartame per person, per year is consumed.[3]

## CAFFEINE

A number of years ago Merle came into my office for some counseling assistance. He was in the auto repair business. In the course of conversation, we talked about his difficulty in sleeping. He also mentioned his struggle with headaches. As we continued to talk, the following information came to light.

Merle was a heavy coffee drinker. I mean *heavy.* Merle would drink up to twenty cups of coffee a day. When he couldn't get coffee, he would drink a number of different soft drinks as a replacement.

The average 6-ounce cup of brewed coffee contains 80–120 mg of caffeine. Instant coffee contains from 66–100 mg. Decaffeinated coffee only contains 2–5 mg. Leaf tea contains 30–80 mg of caffeine. Bag tea contains 42–107 mg, and instant tea contains 30–62 mg. Cocoa contains up to 50 mg of caffeine. Cola drinks contain 15–30 mg of caffeine, and Mountain Dew and Dr. Pepper contain up to 49 mg per 12-ounce glass.

We may know (intellectually) that caffeine is not good for us, but we may continue to put it into our body because we like the taste or the results that immediately occur. To put it into perspective, amounts of more than 250 mg (two to three cups of coffee) can cause some to experience a type of buzzing in their ears. In others it produces insomnia, restlessness, and irritability—and for many, headaches.

What does caffeine do? It is a powerful stimulant that affects the central nervous system. It helps to avert drowsiness and tends to keep people alert. It is used in products like Vivarin and NoDoz. Caffeine is found in weight-loss items like Dexatrim and Appedrine. It is used in menstrual medications like Pre-Mens Forte, Femicin, and Midol. It is found in cold and allergy drugs like Sinarest and Dristan. Caffeine is an item that is found in Excedrin (a headache medication) and other pain relief drugs like Vanquish, Anacin, Bromo-Seltzer, and Empirin.

Coffee specialty houses seem to be popping up in every shopping center. More and more young people are taking up coffee and tea drinking. Flavored coffees can be purchased at many convenience stores. Coffee, tea, and soft drinks are big business. Headaches are also big business.

If caffeine produces headaches, then why is it found in headache medicine? Caffeine helps to constrict blood vessels. This constriction helps to reduce head pain. The problem occurs when the person no longer puts caffeine in their body. The body has an immediate withdrawal reaction. The blood vessels proceed to expand. This causes pain that drives the person to put more caffeine in his body through the means of coffee, tea, sodas, or pain medications that contain caffeine. The person is now caught in a vicious circle. He becomes a caffeine "junky."

Now, back to Merle. I suggested that he might consider reducing his caffeine intake. I made the mistake of not talking to him about his possible withdrawal reactions. Upon his next visit, he told me that he stopped caffeine "cold turkey." This immediate withdrawal of the caffeine stimulant to his body caused him massive nausea, vomiting, terrible headaches, and energy loss.

He said that he was so sick that he couldn't go to work for three days. He then got better, and his headaches disappeared.

Is it best to stop caffeine immediately or slowly withdraw? The answer is, "Yes." Immediate withdrawal speeds up the process and will help reduce headaches quickly. The drawback is that there may be a few days of being uncomfortable. If you withdraw slowly, you will probably eliminate most of the negative withdrawal reactions. The problem is that you might drag out the process of withdrawing from caffeine indefinitely.

For most people, it does not mean that they must *completely* discontinue drinking caffeinated coffee, tea, or soft drinks. It just means that they need to reduce their caffeine intake, which is what is causing their headaches.

There are some researchers who believe that caffeine may be a co-carcinogen that contributes to cancer of the breast, kidney, colon, pancreas, and bladder. Caffeine has a tendency to stimulate excess stomach acid.[4]

### MSG

Heidi loved to eat Chinese food. It was one of her favorite meals. However, Chinese food didn't like Heidi. Often her "great" meals would be followed by great headaches.

Heidi, along with many others, has an explosive reaction to a food additive that is often used in food in Chinese restaurants and many food products. It is called *monosodium glutamate*, or MSG. MSG can cause shivering, nausea, faintness, and headaches.

MSG is found in instant and canned soups, dry-roasted nuts, instant gravies, and frozen dinners. It is also found in self-basting turkeys, some potato chips, and seasonings. Breadcrumbs, croutons, and various salty snacks often contain MSG.

Other possible sources for MSG can be hydrolyzed protein, soy protein, sodium or calcium caseinate, malt extract, and glumatic acid.

Items like gelatin, yeast, and fermented or cultured items can be carriers of MSG.

### CHOCOLATE

Keri loved her chocolate. She liked chocolate bars, chocolate cake, chocolate pie, and chocolate ice cream. Chocolate just simply made Keri feel good, so she thought.

Keri had no idea that chocolate contained caffeine, tyramine, theobromine, and phenylethylamine. (Really, who cares when it tastes so good?) Well, Keri should care because chocolate can trigger her headaches when she eats too much of it.

### FOOD ALLERGIES

Trent was two years of age when he first discovered an extreme allergy to peanuts and other nuts. It was not until his teenage years that he began to get a good handle on avoiding a reaction to nuts. Nuts are hidden in so many different foods. Some of Trent's friends were allergic to things like strawberries, garlic, and carrots.

When Trent would have an allergic reaction, his mouth would first break out in sores. Then his throat would begin to close. Then he would have trouble breathing. Eventually, he would break out in hives all over his body. Not a fun day.

Some people are allergic to dairy products like milk and cheese. Milk products, plums, pineapples, raisins, avocados, onions, bananas, spinach, chocolate, nuts, vinegar, and red wine bother many people and can trigger headaches and other bodily reactions. This is because these foods all contain *amines*. The main amine that affects migraines is tyramine.

Tyramine causes blood vessel expansion and contraction that influences headaches. The amines also stimulate the body's stress hormone system. Tyramine has been associated with nightmares and mind-altering drugs like LSD and psilocybin. Just think about the person who has a reaction to tyramine and eats a late-night pizza with a glass of red wine.

## ALCOHOL

Brandon started drinking in high school and continued to do so during his college years. Now an adult, he is a regular drinker. He would not consider himself an alcoholic; he just likes to get "plastered" every now and then. What he doesn't like are his "hangover headaches."

What causes these types of headaches? The first ingredient is probably tyramine, which is present in the alcohol, especially red wine. This most likely causes the arteries to dilate and create pain. The other ingredients are probably acetaldehyde and acetate, which are breakdown products in the alcohol. Add to this cigarette smoking, lack of sleep, the noise that usually accompanies parties, and maybe nervous tension.

Alcohol also interferes with the function of the liver. The result is that the alcohol causes a hypoglycemic effect on the body, which adds to the hangover problem.

## HOT DOGS

Mark loves hot dogs. He enjoys them at home on the barbecue, at picnics, and especially at baseball games. He has never put together the fact that he always has headaches when he eats them. The thought never crossed his mind, because he enjoys eating them.

Many hot dogs contain preservatives known as *sodium nitrites.* Nitrites cause blood vessels to swell. The swelling of blood vessels can bring on the "hot dog headache."

Nitrites are not only found in hot dogs. They can be found in smoked fish, pork and beans, Spam, oily fish, corned beef, bacon, ham, and various sausages.

## HUNGER

Ramona had spent her time at medical school and was now in her internship at a Philadelphia hospital. She had been working the emergency room for several months. With one emergency after another, Ramona's eating schedule was not normal. When she was hungry, she just couldn't just leave a person with a gunshot wound on the table while she went to a deli and got her favorite sub sandwich.

Ramona found that when she did not eat at a regular time, she would get nagging headaches. People who go on fasting diets for weight loss often experience the same thing. They feel faint (their blood sugar level is low), they may break out in a sweat, and headaches follow. They can also become emotionally sensitive or very cranky and hard to live with.

### ICE CREAM

Skip loved his ice cream. Chocolate chip was his favorite. He would sometimes buy a whole pint and eat it before going to bed. Occasionally he would be so engrossed in a television program that he was not aware of how fast he was eating.

He was soon brought back to reality because of the sharp stinging pain from the "ice cream headache." Anyone who has eaten very much ice cream has experienced this event. It is short-lived but very painful.

I used to tell my friends, "The faster you eat ice cream, the better it tastes." When they would get a headache from their mouth being too cold and the nerve endings responding, I would smile and say, "The pain will go away faster if you take a large, deep breath."

"You're mean," you say. I guess you are right, but I sure had a lot of fun.

### MEDICINE

Amber had been married for a little over a year when she began to notice an increase of headaches. It took her awhile before she saw a relationship between her headaches and the birth control pills she was taking.

Sometimes doctors can neglect to personally inform their patients about the side effects of prescription drugs because of busy schedules and time pressures. Often the patient may only receive a paper listing the cautions. For this reason, it becomes your responsibility to ask intelligent questions about the medications you receive from your doctor or pharmacist. Good questions will help to minimize the needless suffering that comes from being ill informed. This is especially important if you are taking more than one medication at the same time.

The following chart contains a partial list of medications that are known to have the side effects of headaches in some people.

| MEDICATIONS AND HEADACHES | | | |
|---|---|---|---|
| Below is a partial list of medications known to cause headaches in some people. | | | |
| Accutane | Adalat | Advil | Bactrim |
| Capoten | Darvon | Demerol | Doxaphene |
| Indameth | Inderal | Indocin | Isoptin |
| Lopressor | Medipren | Midol | Minipress |
| Motrin | Naprosyn | Nitrogard | Nuprin |
| Orudis | Percocet | Procardia | Propoxycon |
| Rogaine | Roxanol | Serpasil | Sorbitrate |
| Tagamet | Tylox | Vicodin | Voltaren |
| Zantac | | | |

Other medications that can be added to the list are corticosteroids that treat asthma and arthritis, estrogen supplements for birth control, ephedrine for the treatment of bronchitis and emphysema, and a host of other drugs.

### VITAMIN OR MINERAL IMBALANCE

Armando had been noticing an increase in his headaches. He didn't like them but was "toughing" his way through the pain. One day he couldn't stand it any longer. He went to see his doctor.

His doctor explored a number of possible causes for the increase of headaches. Finally, he asked Armando about his diet. He soon found out that Armando was a "meat and potatoes" kind of guy. He didn't eat much in the way of fruits and vegetables. Armando had a vitamin and mineral imbalance. The doctor put him on multivitamins and suggested a change in diet. Soon Armando's headaches began to diminish.

Vitamins and minerals help to improve and protect the immune system in the body. It has long been known that stress has a tendency to deplete vitamin B in the body. It is important to take the entire B vitamin complex. The B vitamins assist in the metabolism of carbohydrates, which help prevent hypoglycemia or low blood sugar. Low blood sugar can be responsible for bringing on headaches. Vitamin $B_6$ is especially important in helping to produce serotonin for the control of headaches.

## YEAST

Tiffany loves any kind of baked goods, including breads, rolls, and her favorite—Krispy Kreme doughnuts. Although she was aware of her increase of headaches, she was not aware that anything baked with yeast can affect head pain. Yeast has tyramine in it.

When yeast is mixed with starch in dough, it breaks down the starch into alcohol. The gases from the alcohol cause dough to rise. Most alcohol evaporates during baking. Dough that is allowed to rise over a longer period breaks down to an acid-producing sourdough. The yeast affects some people more than others. Yeast is involved in most fermentation processes, including alcoholic beverages and yogurts.

Since Tiffany has a reaction to yeast, she would be wise to eat in moderation. She might soon find out that her headaches would also moderate.

Now that we have defined the different types of headaches and established the possible causes, let's move on to discovering all-natural strategies for headache pain and stress relief.

# PART III: HEADACHE RELIEF

CHAPTER 8

# Headache Discovery Guide

*If I have ever made any valuable discoveries, it has been owing more to patient attention, than to any other talent.*[1]

—Sir Isaac Newton

I discussed the five major classifications of headaches. I also gave you scenarios of more than sixty causes of headaches to help you readily identify head pain. Now I will give you a simple tool to help you pinpoint what type of headache you may be experiencing.

I believe the most important issue in solving any problem is to understand what is going on. The "Headache Discovery Guide" is designed to assist you in discovering the circumstances, stresses, and possible triggers for your headaches. This inventory will not only be insightful for you, but it may also be of assistance to any physician or counselor you may visit in the future.

Place a check in all the boxes that best indicate what you experience as a headache sufferer.

☐ 1. I feel a dull, throbbing and steady ache in my head. I feel it behind the eyes, on the side of the head, on the top of the head, or in the back of the head.

☐ 2. My head pain is usually moderate rather than severe.

☐ 3. I feel excessive tightness, stiffness, and tenderness of muscles in the head, neck, and back.

☐ 4. I have a loss of appetite without nausea or vomiting.

☐ 5. I often feel pain on both sides of the head.

☐ 6. My head pain is often accompanied by fatigue.

☐ 7. I am aware that emotional stress and strain often accompany my headaches.

☐ 8. I find myself frowning and clenching my jaws a good deal of the time.

☐ 9. Continuing to work or normal physical activity does not cause an increase of my headache pain.

☐ 10. I experience sinus inflammation and mucous membrane swelling inside my nasal passage during my headache.

☐ 11. I have a colored nasal discharge along with swelling of the nasal passage.

☐ 12. I experience a great deal of nasal drainage that often causes a sore throat.

☐ 13. Foul breath odor accompanies the nasal drainage.

☐ 14. I often feel a dull aching in the frontal part of the head that can become quite intense.

☐ 15. I have a general achy feeling in my muscles.

☐ 16. I have itching and irritated eyes.

☐ 17. I find myself sneezing frequently.

☐ 18. I am usually in an irritable mood.

- ☐ 19. I often have fevers and bacterial infections.
- ☐ 20. I often have a blockage of my nasal airways.
- ☐ 21. When I have headaches, I notice that my face is either very red or very ashen in color.
- ☐ 22. I notice that I yawn a great deal.
- ☐ 23. I struggle with periodic food cravings.
- ☐ 24. I struggle with depression quite a bit.
- ☐ 25. I notice that sometimes I have memory problems.
- ☐ 26. I sometimes have fever and chills that accompany my headaches.
- ☐ 27. I sometimes have cold hands and feet that accompany my headaches.
- ☐ 28. I experience frequent urination during my headaches.
- ☐ 29. I periodically experience constipation that accompanies my headaches.
- ☐ 30. I sometimes have diarrhea that accompanies my headaches.
- ☐ 31. When I have a headache, bright lights bother me greatly.
- ☐ 32. Loud noises seem to make my headache worse.
- ☐ 33. My head pounds and throbs during my headache.
- ☐ 34. Any type of movement, like bending over, greatly increases my head pain.
- ☐ 35. When I get headaches, I feel dizzy and foggy in the head, and I feel as if I might fall down.

☐ 36. A ringing in my ears often accompanies my headaches.

☐ 37. Sometimes I feel numbness in my tongue and lips.

☐ 38. The top of my head is sore to touch.

☐ 39. I find that I have trouble concentrating during my headaches.

☐ 40. During my headaches I become anxious, irritable, restless, agitated, or angry.

☐ 41. Because of my headaches, I feel dejected, I desire to withdraw, and sometimes I experience despair.

☐ 42. My headaches cause a sudden and excruciating pain behind or around the eye on one side of the head.

☐ 43. My head pain radiates to the temple, jaw, nose, teeth, and chin.

☐ 44. During my headache, my eyelid on one side begins to droop.

☐ 45. During my headache, my eyes begin to tear up and water.

☐ 46. During my headache, my face becomes flush.

☐ 47. During my headache, my nose begins to congest.

☐ 48. During my headache, I find myself sweating.

☐ 49. When I bend over or move my head from side to side, my head pain increases dramatically.

☐ 50. Since I had my accident, I have more headaches.

☐ 51. I find that stuffy rooms seem to bring on my headaches.

☐ 52. I get headaches when I cough a lot.

- ☐ 53. I am dealing with a medical condition that brings on headaches.
- ☐ 54. Headaches seem to come when I do not get the proper sleep.
- ☐ 55. I get headaches when I exercise too strenuously.
- ☐ 56. I get headaches whenever I have a fever.
- ☐ 57. I get headaches during my menstrual period.
- ☐ 58. I get headaches from car sickness or certain amusement park rides.
- ☐ 59. I get headaches as a result of a neck injury.
- ☐ 60. Whenever I sit or stand for long periods, I get headaches.
- ☐ 61. I sometimes experience headaches after sexual intercourse.
- ☐ 62. Shopping in stores for long periods brings on headaches.
- ☐ 63. I sometimes experience headaches resulting from sporting activities.
- ☐ 64. I get headaches when I don't wear my glasses.
- ☐ 65. I find that I get headaches on the weekends.
- ☐ 66. I get headaches from grinding my teeth together.
- ☐ 67. Chewing a lot of gum gives me headaches.
- ☐ 68. A soreness in my jaw brings about headaches.
- ☐ 69. An abscessed tooth will give me a headache.
- ☐ 70. When my allergies flare up, I get headaches.
- ☐ 71. Sometimes a change in the weather brings about headaches.

- ☐ 72. Smoggy conditions tend to give me headaches.
- ☐ 73. Bright lights or glare from the sun gives me headaches.
- ☐ 74. I get headaches whenever I travel to high altitudes.
- ☐ 75. Loud, blaring noises gives me headaches.
- ☐ 76. The smell of paint thinner or gasoline gives me a headache.
- ☐ 77. Smoky rooms give me headaches.
- ☐ 78. Toxic odors and even some perfumes give me headaches.
- ☐ 79. Whenever I get angry, I seem to get a headache.
- ☐ 80. When I have excessive worry or anxiety, I get headaches.
- ☐ 81. Broken or damaged relationships bother me a great deal and bring about headaches.
- ☐ 82. The stress of change can cause me to have a headache.
- ☐ 83. The pressures of child rearing often cause me headaches.
- ☐ 84. I find that headaches often accompany my depression.
- ☐ 85. Making very important decisions is difficult and sometimes causes headaches.
- ☐ 86. Concerns over finances often give rise to headaches.
- ☐ 87. Excessive concern about personal or family health issues can generate headaches.
- ☐ 88. Going through difficult marital problems brings on headaches.

- ☐ 89. Crisis or trauma situations cause me to have headaches.
- ☐ 90. I often get headaches because of my difficult working conditions.
- ☐ 91. I get headaches at school because of difficult relationships and scholastic demands on me.
- ☐ 92. My schedule is so demanding that I am overloaded, and it causes headaches.
- ☐ 93. I get headaches from drinking too many diet soft drinks.
- ☐ 94. I get headaches from drinking too much coffee or tea.
- ☐ 95. When I eat Chinese food, I get headaches.
- ☐ 96. I love chocolate, but I get headaches after eating it.
- ☐ 97. I am allergic to certain foods that bring about headaches.
- ☐ 98. I get headaches after drinking alcoholic beverages.
- ☐ 99. I seem to get headaches after eating hot dogs or lunch meats.
- ☐ 100. When I eat ice cream too fast, I get headaches.
- ☐ 101. Some of the medications that I take seem to cause me headaches.

- Statements 1–9 relate to *tension* headaches.
- Statements 10–20 relate to *sinus* headaches.
- Statements 21–41 relate to *migraine* headaches.
- Statements 42–49 relate to *cluster* headaches.
- Statements 50–101 relate to *mixed* headaches.
- Statements 50–65 are *physical* causes for headaches.
- Statements 66–69 are *dental* causes for headaches.

- Statements 70–78 are *environmental* causes for headaches.
- Statements 79–92 are *emotional* causes for headaches.
- Statements 93–101 are *food and medicine* causes for headaches.

My headaches tend to lean more toward:

☐ Tension ☐ Sinus ☐ Migraine ☐ Cluster ☐ Mixed

I first started experiencing headaches when

..........................................................................................................................

..........................................................................................................................

..........................................................................................................................

..........................................................................................................................

Was there any massive change, crisis, or trauma associated with the beginning of your headaches? If so, can you describe the events?

..........................................................................................................................

..........................................................................................................................

..........................................................................................................................

..........................................................................................................................

How many times a week do you experience headaches?

..........................................................................................................................

..........................................................................................................................

..........................................................................................................................

..........................................................................................................................

Have you had any recent increase or decrease of headaches?

.......................................................................................................................

How would you describe your headache pain?

.......................................................................................................................

.......................................................................................................................

.......................................................................................................................

.......................................................................................................................

How do others around you (family, friends, and fellow workers) respond to your headaches?

.......................................................................................................................

.......................................................................................................................

.......................................................................................................................

.......................................................................................................................

Do your headaches (even though painful) have a positive gain for you in some way? Do you get extra attention? Do your headaches get you out of work or situations you don't like, or can you, in a sense, get even with someone by having them? Describe possible positive gains from your headaches.

.......................................................................................................................

.......................................................................................................................

.......................................................................................................................

.......................................................................................................................

Your headache pain might be trying to tell you something. What might be the possible message?

.......................................................................................................................

................................................................................................................................

................................................................................................................................

................................................................................................................................

How would you describe your general feeling tone at this time in your life? Complete the following sentences.

Right now I feel...

................................................................................................................................

................................................................................................................................

................................................................................................................................

................................................................................................................................

I would like to see the following changes in my life at this time:

................................................................................................................................

................................................................................................................................

................................................................................................................................

................................................................................................................................

Do you have hurts in your life other than your hurting headaches?

Hurts from your parents?

................................................................................................................................

Hurts from your elementary school years?

................................................................................................................................

Hurts from your junior high school years?

................................................................................................................................

Hurts from your high school years?

..............................................................................................................

Hurts from your adult life?

..............................................................................................................

Do you feel that you are under a lot of stress at this time in your life? What are the stressors that you are facing right now?

..............................................................................................................

..............................................................................................................

..............................................................................................................

..............................................................................................................

| DISCOMFORT CHART | | |
|---|---|---|
| Circle the words that describe the pain and discomfort you feel at this time. | | |
| Abominable | Excruciating | Racking |
| Aggravating | Exhausting | Radiating |
| Annoying | Gnawing | Searing |
| Blinding | Grating | Shooting |
| Burning | Horrible | Stabbing |
| Constant | Intense | Terrible |
| Crushing | Irritating | Throbbing |
| Debilitating | Miserable | Tormenting |
| Distressing | Nagging | Unbearable |
| Disturbing | Pulverizing | Unending |
| Exasperating | Punishing | Unpleasant |

Stress can take on many forms. Physical stress can come from accidents, exercise, postural misalignment, sports, or just plain hard work. Environmental stress can be caused by noise, weather, altitude, and toxic chemicals. Medicines, food allergies, diet, and common caffeine in coffee, tea, or soft drinks can trigger biochemical stress. Emotional stress can be created from misunderstanding, broken relationships, tragedy, negative emotions, or a change in habits.

Dr. Thomas Holmes and Dr. Richard Rahe developed what is called the Holmes & Rahe Stress Test. It measures the number of changes in a person's life and gives them a total stress score rating. A large amount of stress can bring about headaches in many people.[2]

In the following chart, indicate how many times a particular change has occurred in your life during the past twelve months. Multiply the number of occurrences times the stress value listed. Then total all of the scores to get your total life-change value, or more practically, the amount of stress you are facing at this time as a result of the changes you indicated.[3]

| LIFE EVENT | OCCURRENCES | STRESS VALUE | YOUR SCORE |
|---|---|---|---|
| Death of a spouse | | 100 | |
| Divorce | | 73 | |
| Marital separation | | 65 | |
| Detention in jail | | 63 | |
| Death of close family member | | 63 | |
| Major personal injury or illness | | 53 | |
| Marriage | | 50 | |

| LIFE EVENT | OCCURRENCES | STRESS VALUE | YOUR SCORE |
|---|---|---|---|
| Being fired from work | | 47 | |
| Marital reconciliation | | 45 | |
| Retirement from work | | 47 | |
| Major change in health or behavior of family member | | 44 | |
| Pregnancy | | 40 | |
| Sexual difficulties | | 39 | |
| Gaining a new family member by birth, adoption, moving in | | 39 | |
| Major business readjustment reorganization, bankruptcy | | 39 | |
| Major change in financial status—better or worse | | 38 | |
| Death of close friend | | 37 | |
| Changing to different line of work | | 36 | |
| Major change in arguments with spouse—more or less | | 35 | |
| Mortgage greater than $10,000 | | 31 | |
| Foreclosure on mortgage or loan | | 30 | |
| Major change in responsibilities at work—promotion or demotion | | 29 | |
| Son or daughter leaving home: marriage, attending school | | 29 | |
| Trouble with in-laws | | 29 | |

| LIFE EVENT | OCCURRENCES | STRESS VALUE | YOUR SCORE |
|---|---|---|---|
| Outstanding personal achievement | | 28 | |
| Wife begins or ceases work | | 26 | |
| Beginning or ending school | | 26 | |
| Major change in living conditions | | 25 | |
| Revision of personal habits | | 24 | |
| Troubles with boss | | 23 | |
| Change in work hours / conditions | | 20 | |
| Change in residence | | 20 | |
| Changing to a new school | | 20 | |
| Change in recreation—more / less | | 19 | |
| Change in church activities | | 19 | |
| Change in social activities | | 18 | |
| Mortgage or loan under $10,000 | | 17 | |
| Change in sleeping habits | | 16 | |
| Change in family get-togethers | | 15 | |
| Change in eating habits | | 15 | |
| Vacation | | 13 | |

| LIFE EVENT | OCCURRENCES | STRESS VALUE | YOUR SCORE |
|---|---|---|---|
| Christmas | | 12 | |
| Minor violations of the law | | 11 | |
| YOUR TOTAL LIFE CHANGE OR TOTAL STRESS LEVEL SCORE | | | |

- Scores of 150–199: 37 percent likely to encounter illness in the near future
- Scores of 200–299: 50 percent likely to encounter illness in the near future
- Scores of 300 or more: 80 percent likely to encounter illness in the near future

## HEADACHE DIARY

Headaches are not a disease or an illness. They are a symptom of something else going on in the body. Headaches have a cause-and-effect relationship. Something causes the headache to emerge. Something triggers the body to respond with head pain. Part of seeking to find headache relief involves keeping an accurate diary of your headache pattern. This diary will then begin to help you discover the cause, or causes, that bring about your headaches.

**LEVEL OF PAIN**

| LITTLE | MILD | MODERATE | STRONG | SEVERE |
|---|---|---|---|---|
| ← | | | | → |
| 1 2 | 3 4 | 5 6 | 7 8 | 9 10 |

| DATE OF HEADACHE | TIME OF DAY | LEVEL OF PAIN | DURATION OF PAIN | POSSIBLE TRIGGERS | CIRCUMSTANCES SURROUNDING—AND/OR THOUGHTS/FEELINGS |
|---|---|---|---|---|---|
| | | | | | |
| | | | | | |
| | | | | | |
| | | | | | |
| | | | | | |
| | | | | | |
| | | | | | |
| | | | | | |
| | | | | | |
| | | | | | |
| | | | | | |
| | | | | | |
| | | | | | |

| DATE OF HEADACHE | TIME OF DAY | LEVEL OF PAIN | DURATION OF PAIN | POSSIBLE TRIGGERS | CIRCUMSTANCES SURROUNDING—AND/OR THOUGHTS/FEELINGS |
|---|---|---|---|---|---|
| | | | | | |
| | | | | | |
| | | | | | |
| | | | | | |
| | | | | | |
| | | | | | |
| | | | | | |
| | | | | | |
| | | | | | |

Once the causes, or triggers, for your headaches are known, then you can work on reducing or minimizing those causes. You will not be able to completely eliminate headaches entirely because there are too many complex factors, such as our lifestyles and environment. But you will be able to lower the frequency and the severity of your headaches with drug-free strategies.

CHAPTER 9

# Drug-Free Strategies for Headache Relief

*If we could give every individual the right amount of nourishment and exercise, not too little and not too much, we would have found the safest way to health.*[1]

—HIPPOCRATES

Headaches are a symptom of some circumstance or factor in an individual's life. These circumstances or factors act as triggers to set off or create the head pain. In some cases, the headache can arise from a single factor like drinking too much alcohol and getting the "hangover" headache. In most cases, headaches come from a combination of factors that build up to the point where they spill over and produce a headache. An individual who is in poor health, under a great deal of stress at work, having marital problems and financial difficulties, experiencing allergies, and taking heavy medications may not be able to escape headaches.

The causes or triggers for headaches fall into four major categories:

1. *Physical.* This includes things like sinus problems, dental difficulties, accidents, brain tumor,

breathing issues, sleep disturbances, fever, motion sickness, menstrual periods, body alignment, sports injuries, vision issues, illness and disease, and so on.

2. *Ingestion.* This includes things like too much caffeine, food allergies, alcohol, eating Chinese food, chemicals in foods, various medications, and so on.
3. *Psychological.* This includes things like negative thinking, anger, anxiety, broken relationships, major decisions, depression, crisis and trauma, excessive change, stress and overload, and so on.
4. *Environment.* This includes things like changes in the weather, exposure to toxic chemicals, fumes and perfume, allergies from dust and pollen, excessive noise, glare, high altitude, and so on.

In many books on headaches, a large portion of the discussion revolves around the explanation of how head pain is created. Often there is a great deal of focus on *serotonin,* a chemical produced by the body.

The human nervous system is made up of cells called *neurons.* Neurons have a nucleus surrounded by cytoplasm. Most neurons have single long fibers known as *axons.* The axons have branches extending off called *dendrites.* Nerves can be single, or they can be gathered into bunches. The body has several billion neurons that are all connected to each other sending messages back and forth.

Nerves carry impulses or messages from the brain to various parts of the body. My brain sends messages down my arms, to my fingers, to type on a computer to produce this book on headaches.

Nerves can also send messages from various parts of the body back to the brain. If I touch something hot, the message is sent from my fingers back to my brain. My brain then sends a return message back to my fingers to remove them from the hot surface. "Hello. Your hand is burning!"

The nervous system is made up of three major divisions. The first is the *central nervous system.* This includes the brain and spinal cord that runs down the back. The second is the *peripheral nervous system.* This involves nerve branches extending off of the central nervous system. These nerves carry messages back and forth from the body to the central nervous system. The third is the *autonomic nervous system.* This is made up of nerves that regulate all of the involuntary processes of the body such as breathing and pumping of the heart.

The place where axons connect to dendrites is called a *synapse.* When messages or impulses transfer from the axon to the dendrite, the process is made possible by a chemical substance called *serotonin.* Serotonin is a neurotransmitter. It influences the cardiovascular, renal, immune, and gastrointestinal systems. It is also partly involved in the regulating of mood in an individual.

Medical science believes (although they don't quite know how) that a disruption of the synthesis, metabolism, or uptake of serotonin plays a part in schizophrenia, depression, compulsive disorders, learning problems, and headaches. People with these problems seem to have a reduction of serotonin. Because of this, pharmaceutical companies are attempting to produce drugs that will affect the production of serotonin.

Most of the discussions regarding serotonin circle around the production—or lack of it—in the body. Very little research is being done on *why* there is a disruption in the first place. Does serotonin disruption cause the mood change, or does the mood change cause the disruption of serotonin?

I am of the belief that the mood change (caused by the thinking—the reception and perception process in the body) is responsible for the disruption of the serotonin.

We have a good example of this when it comes to a chemical in the body called *adrenaline*. Adrenaline is a hormone produced in the adrenal glands. Its job is to excite and create extra alertness and energy to help in times of fight or flight.

Adrenaline is produced whenever there is a real or perceived stress or emergency.

When you are crossing the street and a large truck is about to hit you, the perceived danger, or stress, triggers the instant production of adrenaline. As adrenaline rushes through your body, it helps give you the strength and energy to jump out of the way. Once you are safe, you can still feel the effects of the adrenaline. Your heart will be beating fast. You will be breathing hard, and your body will be shaking a little from the extra surge of energy. After a period, your body will relax—adrenaline will drain off—and you will return to a normal state.

Now, let's ask the question: did the adrenaline cause the perception of danger, or did the perception of danger cause the adrenaline to flow? Of course, we know the answer. It was the perception of danger, or the reality of danger, that triggered the production of adrenaline.

I believe that the change or disruption of serotonin in the body is caused by real or perceived stressors and circumstances. I don't believe the serotonin is responsible for the stress or the mood change.

I now have a choice. Do I attempt to regulate the serotonin by the use of chemicals and drugs—and ignore the stressors that may be the cause? Or do I attempt to regulate the stressors and circumstances—and eliminate the need for drugs and chemicals? Drugs and chemicals have a place, but they should not be the primary focus. They only temporarily mask or cover the real cause of the problem, which we will discuss later. For now, we will begin to direct our attention toward the nondrug treatment of headaches.

CHAPTER 10

# Physical Strategies for Headache Relief

*The poorest man would not part with health for money, but the richest would gladly part with all his money for health.*[1]

—C. C. Colton

To stimulate the release of endorphins for the relief of headaches, various acupressure points can be massaged. There are several different massage techniques that can be used. They are illustrated below.

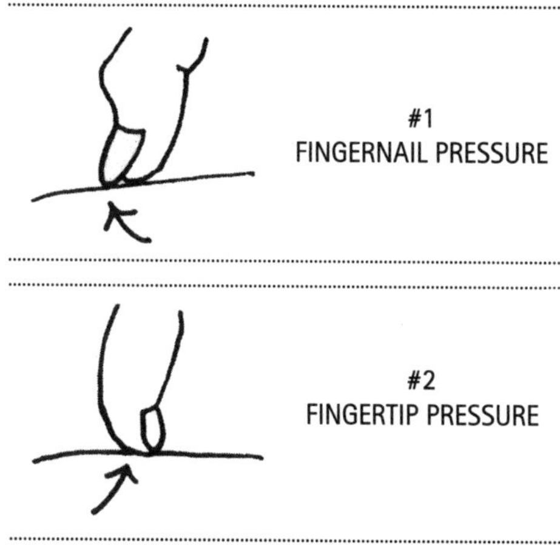

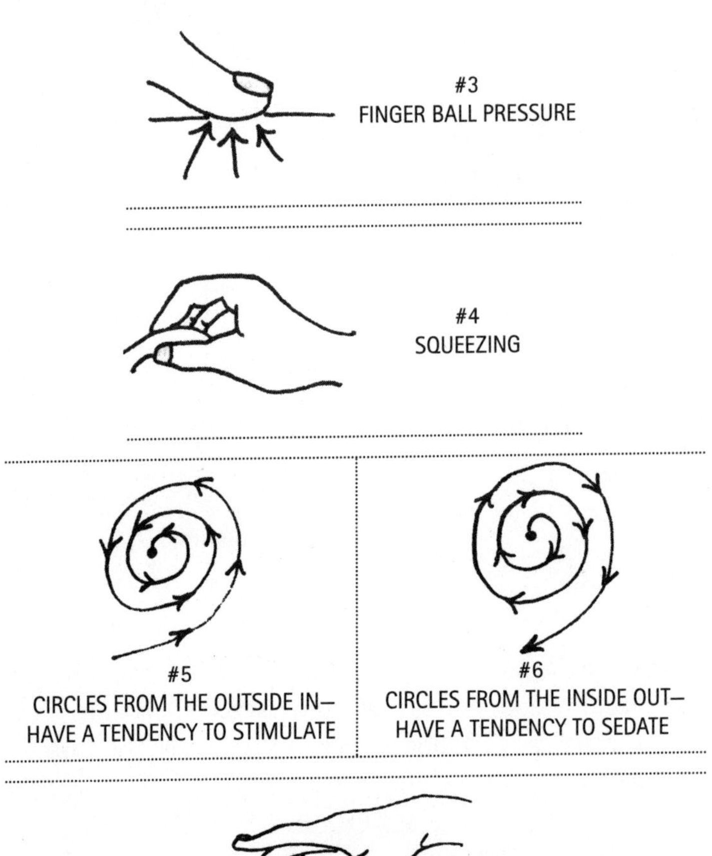

#3
FINGER BALL PRESSURE
#4
SQUEEZING
#5
CIRCLES FROM THE OUTSIDE IN—
HAVE A TENDENCY TO STIMULATE
#6
CIRCLES FROM THE INSIDE OUT—
HAVE A TENDENCY TO SEDATE
#7
WHEN MASSAGING, THE CIRCULAR MOTION SHOULD BE FAIRLY RAPID,
ABOUT 2 TO 3 CYCLES PER SECOND.


The amount of time can range from thirty seconds to five minutes, depending on the location. When applying direct pressure, it may last from thirty seconds to one minute on each location. Do not be surprised if you, or the person you might be helping, feel a reduction of pain in as little as fifteen seconds.

The massaging, or direct pressure, will not be as effective on people who have just eaten a meal. It is best to wait an hour or more in those cases. The pressure points will also not be as effective with someone who is drinking iced or alcoholic beverages or eating spicy or sour foods. Common sense will tell you not to massage on open wounds, recent scars, or where there is infection. Do not use these pressure points on pregnant women or anyone with serious cardiac problems. Discontinue if the symptoms become aggravated.

One of the main acupressure points is found in the webbing between your thumb and your first finger. Start with this acupressure point first. When the thumb and index finger are squeezed together, the acupressure point can be found by pressing hard on the highest point of the muscle with your free thumb. When you press hard, you will find it to be very painful. If it is not painful, you do not have the right spot. Move around until you find the most painful spot.

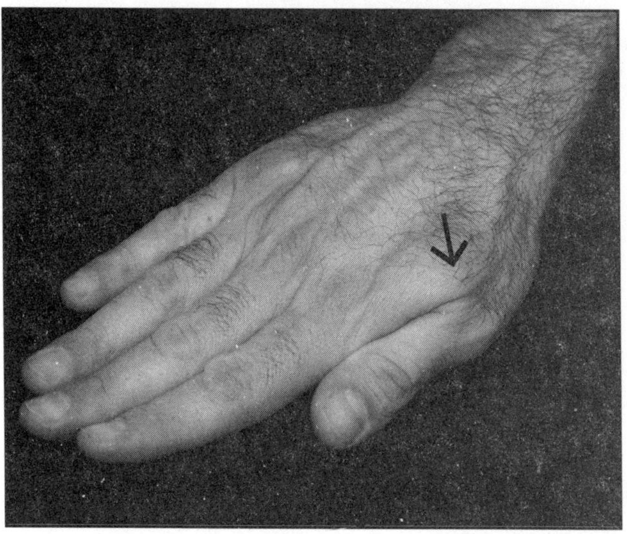

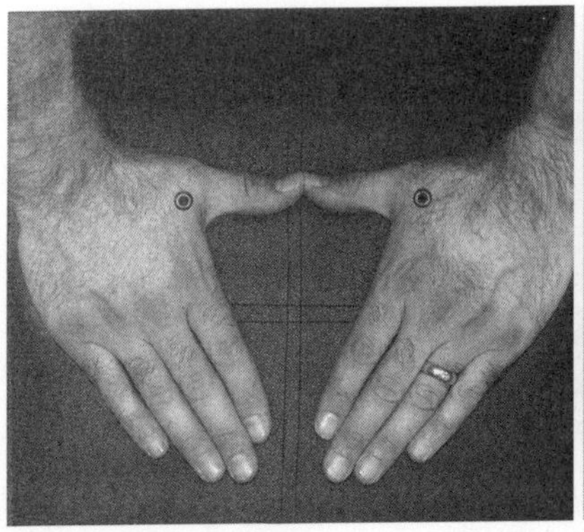

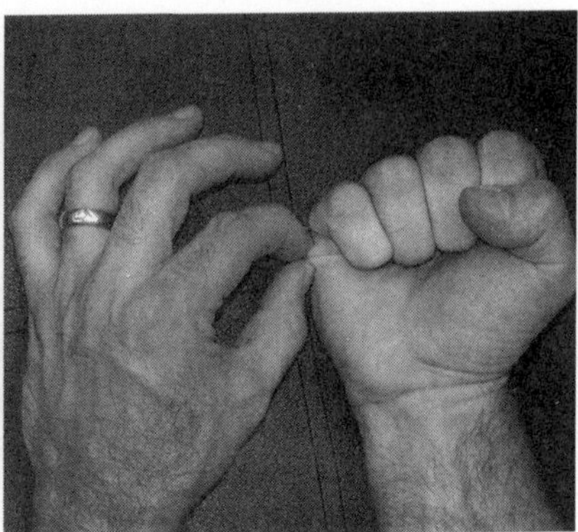

After massaging the point in the webbing of the hands, move to point located on the inside part of the wrist. This acupressure point will not be painful at all. Massage for about twenty to thirty seconds. It is even better if you could have someone help you by massaging both points in the webbing of the hands and both wrists at the same time.

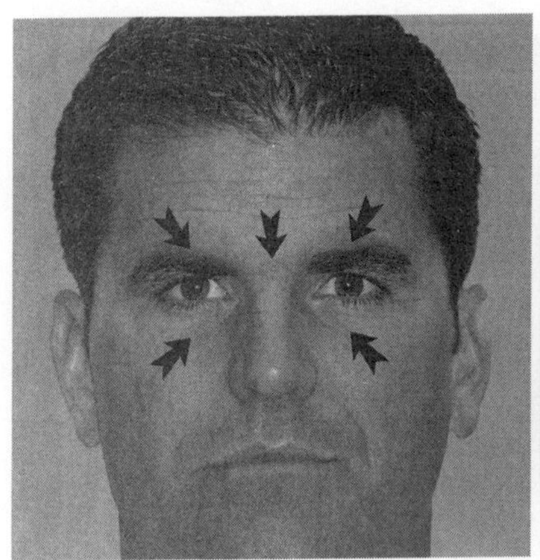

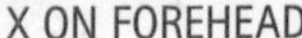

X ON FOREHEAD

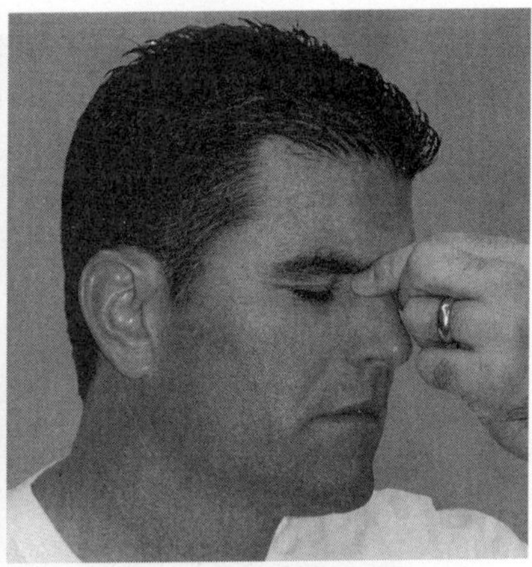

SQUEEZING FROM SIDE

The third acupressure spot is located between your eyebrows. It can be stimulated by squeezing the area between your thumb and index finger and pressing inward at the same time. It can also be stimulated by pressing straight in with pressure and massaging around in circles. Then press and squeeze the area where the top of the bridge of your nose and your eyebrows come together. This will often be a tender area that is caused by muscles being in tension.

Squeeze and push this area for about thirty seconds. Then squeeze for the count of three and relax for the count of three...squeeze and relax...squeeze and relax. Keep doing this for another thirty seconds.

The fourth major acupressure points for headaches are located in the back of the head. These points are especially helpful for tension headaches, but they are a little hard to find.

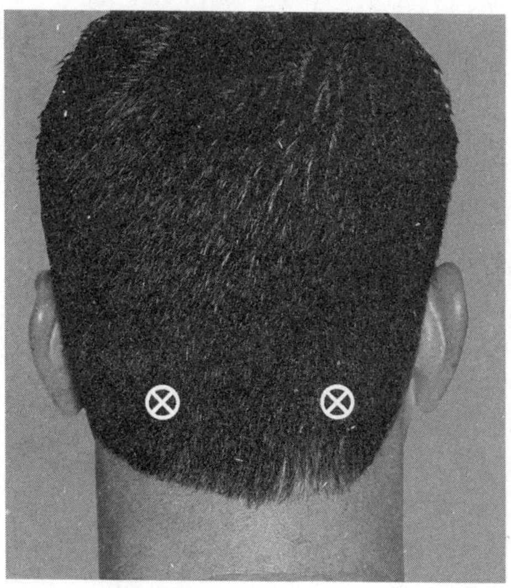

Take both of your middle fingers and place each one on the point of the bone just below each earlobe. Slowly move your fingers back, around, and up the bone until they slip into the notch where the bone above the neckline is. Now, press firmly with your fingers; at the same time push your head backwards. Massage this point for about thirty seconds. Some pain will be felt in this location.

Certain acupressure points when massaged will be more painful than others. This is normal. When people first massage the painful points, they have a tendency to not massage very hard because of the pain. When they massage lightly, they lose the effectiveness of the stimulation. The pressure that is to be applied is about ten to fifteen pounds—fairly strong. The pain should be somewhere between moderate to high but not quite to severe pain. In a simple word, it will be just a little uncomfortable. When that occurs, you will be applying the right amount of pressure.

The fifth major acupressure point is located on the side of the head. This point can be found by placing your two index fingers on the bone at the outside corners of your eyes. As you move your fingers slowly back toward your ears, you will notice there is a ridge of bone. It runs from the corner of your eyes back toward your ears.

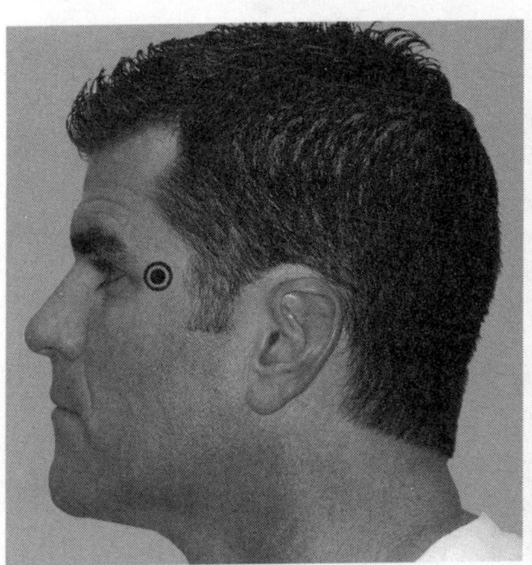

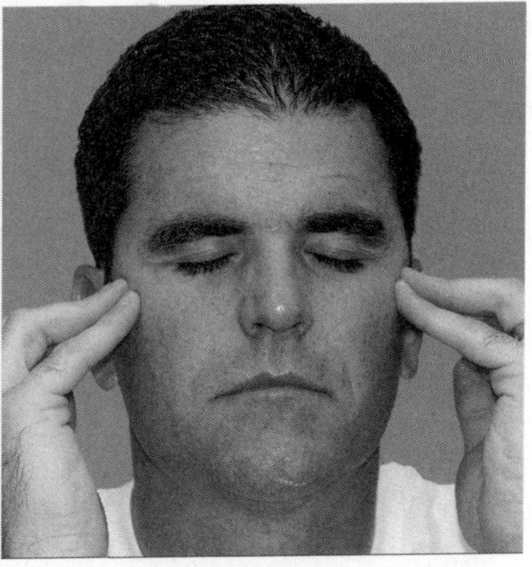

Place the balls of all four fingers of each hand on the top of the ridge of this bone. Press down firmly on this ridge, and vigorously move your fingers back and forth on the ridge. Continue this motion for about twenty seconds. Keep your eyes closed during the massaging. When you stop, keep your eyes closed until the sensation slows down, and then slowly open them.

There are a number of other acupressure points that have been found helpful for the release of headache pain. The points listed below should be massaged for about thirty seconds or more. Each person varies a little, and some points work better for some than others. Experiment with the different points to find out what is best for you.

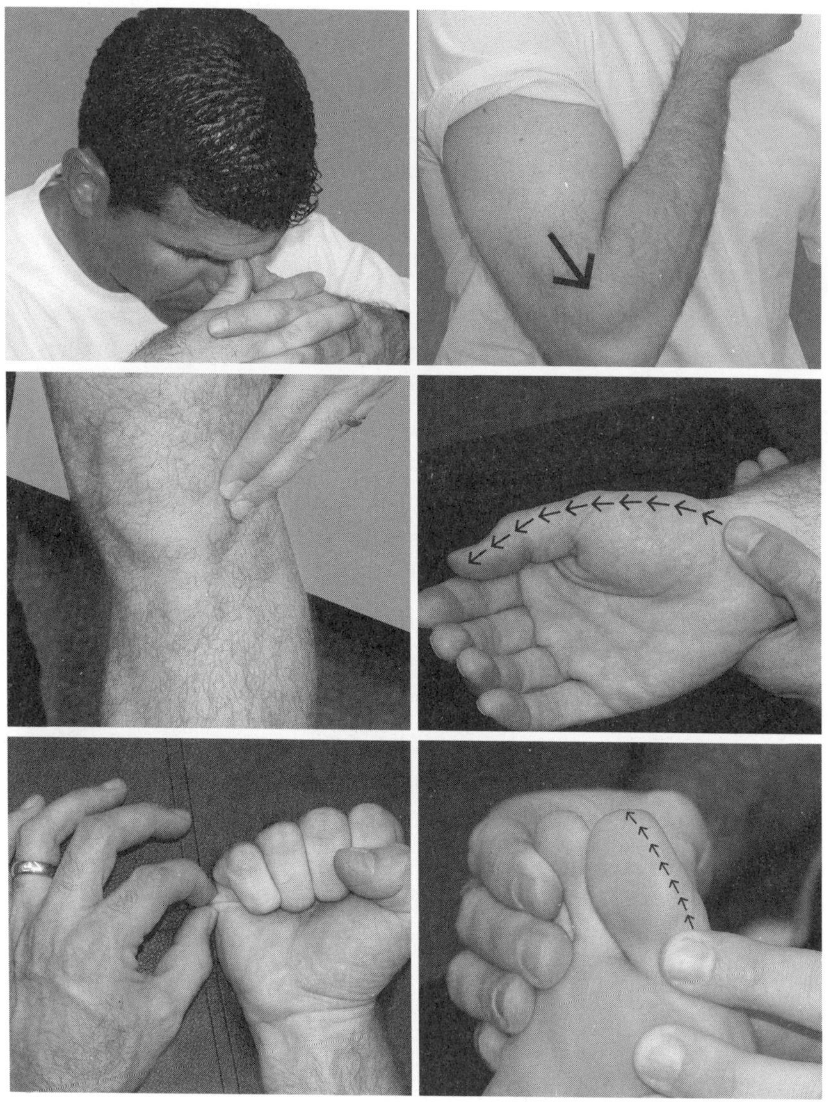

## ALIGNMENT AND POSTURE

The human body has been wonderfully designed for motion. The skeletal system helps keep the body erect and upright. The muscular system pulls bones back and forth to walk, run, turn, pick up things, and put down things. Muscles are divided into two basic types. Static muscles primarily regulate posture and help fight against the pull of gravity. This would include some of the muscles of the neck, back, hips, legs, and feet. These muscles help to control the movement of the load-bearing joints of the shoulders, hips, knees, and ankles. Phasic muscles are primarily designed for strength and activity. These would include muscles like the biceps, triceps, and quadriceps.

When we strain static muscles, or if they are used incorrectly, phasic muscles will take over the job. It is not long before the phasic muscles get tired of the strain, and pain and stiffness follow. The pain arises because there is a reduction of oxygen to the muscles and an inability of the muscles to burn sugar properly. This inability to burn sugar properly produces lactic acid. As lactic acid increases—so does pain in the muscles.

To assist in the removal of lactic acid and the proper burning of sugar, oxygen input is extremely important. Many people unconsciously breathe in a very shallow manner. There is little oxygen intake.

## TAKE A DEEP BREATH

Take a moment and become aware of your own breathing. Is it shallow, or is it deep? When you run or exercise vigorously, you naturally begin to breathe deeper. Your body is crying for extra oxygen to help break down the sugar, which is necessary for the energy you are expending. Shallow breathing will not help to get rid of pain.

Take the simple act of crying. It involves the tightening of muscles of the chest, neck, stomach, and face. Breathing is usually shallow. If you take deep breaths when you first start to cry, it will slow down the physical crying process. Physical or emotional pain may still be present, but deep breaths help to relax the body when it becomes stressed.

### PAIN IS TRYING TO TELL YOU SOMETHING

Pain in a particular part of the body is sending a message to the brain. It is saying that what we are doing is not beneficial—it is a warning signal. What is the usual pattern of behavior for dealing with the pain we feel? Our first tendency is to try and ignore the pain message. Then when it continues, we try to get rid of it with the use of stimulants or pain-killing drugs. When that doesn't work, we turn to surgery in an attempt to obliterate the pain.

Seldom does the person ask, "Why am I feeling this pain? What am I doing to cause this pain? What is happening to me that's contributing to the pain I am feeling?" Instead, we reach for alcohol or some pills to help mask, cover, or soothe the pain. Thus, when the effect of the alcohol, pills, or even surgery diminishes—the pain returns. *Hello. Maybe there is a reason for all the pain.*

Again, take a moment and become aware of your own body. Is it sending any messages to you right now? Are you feeling any pain? Have you been frowning? What would happen if you consciously attempted to relax the muscles of your forehead and in between your eyes? Do you feel tightness in your jaw muscles? Can you relax them? As you slowly move your head from side to side, or from front to back, do you sense any neck pain? Are you aware of any pain in your upper or lower back? Do your legs or feet ache?

Even as I write these words, I am aware of some strain on my own lower back. Pain messages are being sent to my brain. What are they trying to say? Should I ignore them and take an aspirin? Or should I listen to them say to me, "You have been sitting in your chair for a long time typing on this book. You need to get up—do some stretching—and move around a little. Your body needs some movement, some exercise." Well, I am going to listen to my body. I am going to get up and do some stretching exercises before I continue writing the next paragraph.

Stress and strain in the back and neck can help lead to headaches. Where do the stress and strain come from? Naturally, some comes from the pressure and demands of our high-paced society. Some of the tightening of the muscles is a result of how we view life and the various people with whom we come in contact. If we have a difficult boss to work for, we may be frustrated and angry. It may be causing muscle contractions in our body. That's where the word *uptight* comes from. Often muscle strain comes from our posture and body alignment—or better—our misalignment.

## PAIN FREE

How we sit, walk, and stand has a great influence on our body either for good or for bad. In his book *Pain Free: A Revolutionary Method for Stopping Chronic Pain,* Pete Egoscue says, "I have never known a migraine sufferer whose head, neck, and shoulders were not out of position in the characteristic mode of forward flexion."[2] Mr. Egoscue is an anatomical physiologist. In his clinic in San Diego, he has treated some of the most famous names in sports and business.

Mr. Egoscue has helped many people with ankle, knee, back, shoulder, and neck pain injury. He helps them to avoid surgery as a solution. He, in turn, suggests that their pain may be caused by their body misalignment. When that is corrected, there is no need for surgery, and the pain diminishes.

At the Egoscue Method Clinic they recommend the following exercises to help eliminate headaches caused by alignment dysfunctions. These exercises are very simple to do and only take about twenty minutes. They suggest that the exercises be done in the morning. They also advise that the exercises be continued after the pain has been relieved as a preventive measure to future pain.

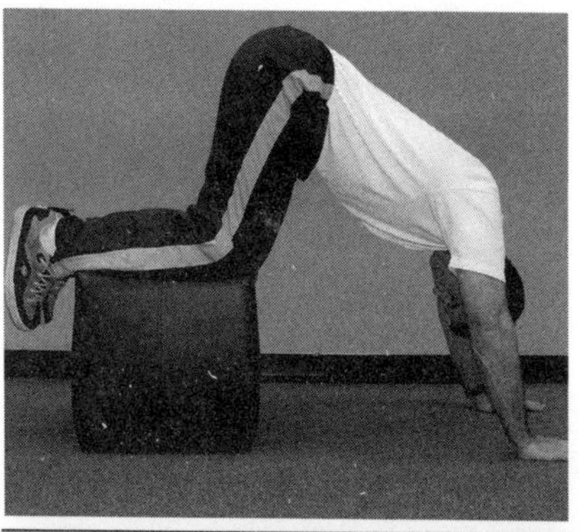

*Static extension*

- Relax head toward floor.
- Your back is arched down.
- Keep elbows straight.
- Hips are ahead of knees about 6–8 inches.
- Hold for one minute to begin with—build up to two minutes.

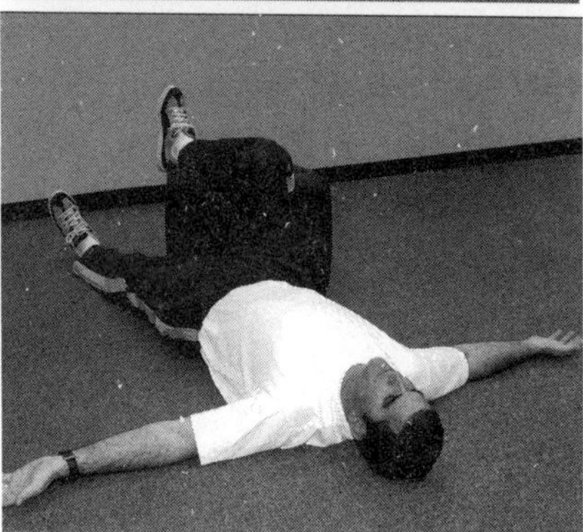

*Static back*

- Lie on back—legs bent at right angles to chair.
- Rest hands on floor, palms up or on stomach.
- Breathe from diaphragm, using stomach muscles.
- Hold position for five to ten minutes.

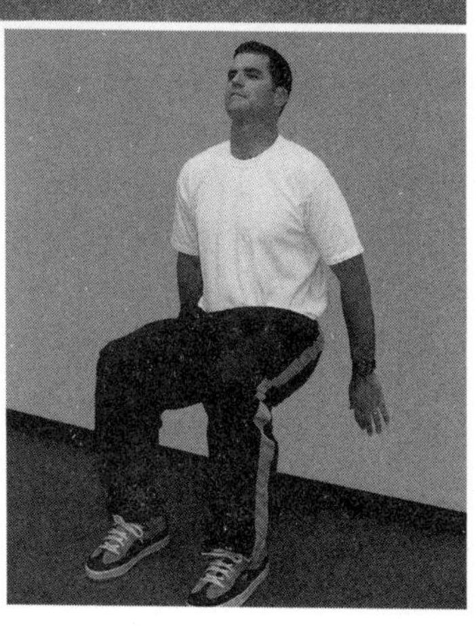

*Air bench*

- Stand with back against wall.
- Walk feet forward and slide down at same time.
- Knees are over ankles in 90-degree sitting position.
- Hold position for one to three minutes.
- Walk around after doing the exercise.

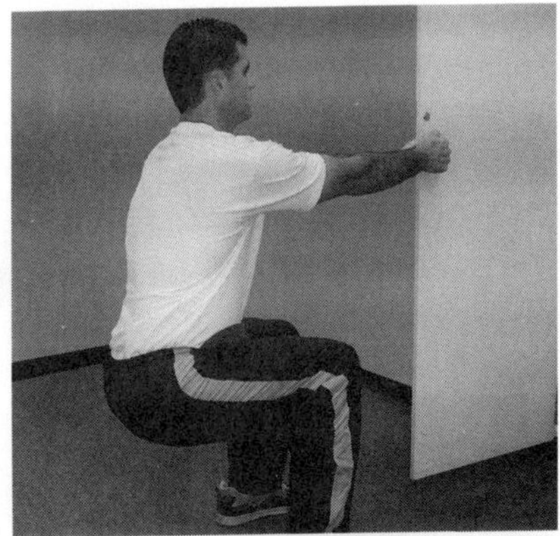

*Squat*

- Hold on to object.
- Arms are straight.
- Knees and hips are parallel—and aligned with feet.
- Keep torso straight with head over hips.
- Hold position for one to two minutes.

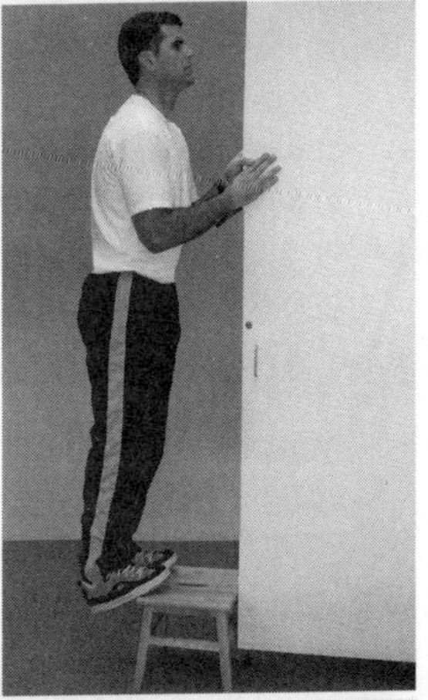

*Gravity drop*

- Stand on a step or block.
- Feet are shoulder width apart—pointing straight ahead.
- Hold on with hands for balance.
- Let weight press into heels.
- Hold one to three minutes.

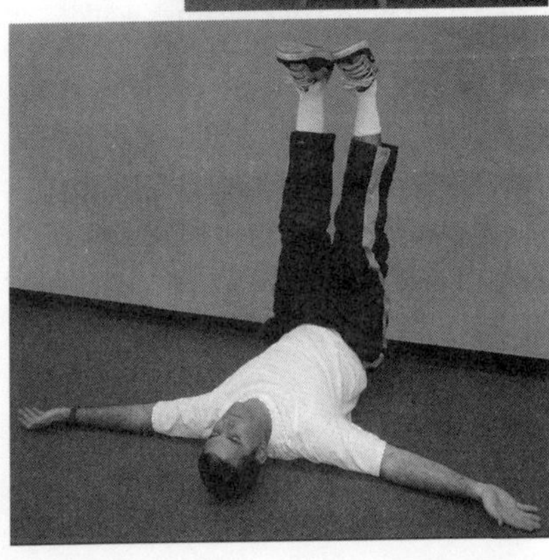

*Static wall*

- Lie on back—feet straight up against wall—hip-width apart.
- Bottom is close to wall.
- Tighten thighs.
- Flex feet toward floor.
- Hold position for three to five minutes.

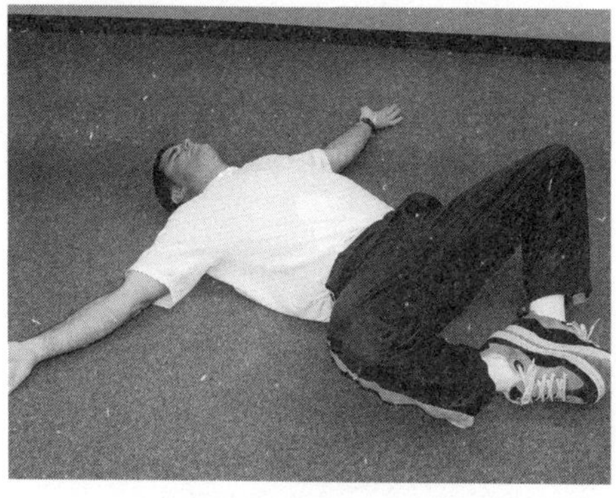

*Frog*

- Lie on back—feet drawn up, with soles touching each other.
- Relax.
- Do not press down on knees.
- You should not feel pain in your back.
- Hold position for one minute.

## THE BODY TALKS—DO YOU LISTEN?

The human body often mirrors through the muscles and organs what is going on in the thinking process. This is illustrated by an interesting study done by W. J. Grace and D. T. Graham. They studied 128 patients in a hospital outpatient department. The interviews lasted about one hour and took place as often as twice a week. Twelve symptoms or diseases were studied. The following results were discovered.[3]

1. *Urticaria (hives), 31 patients*—occurred when the individual saw himself as being mistreated. He felt he was receiving a blow, and there was nothing he could do about it. "I was taking a beating" and "My fiancée hit me, but what could I do?" were typical statements.

2. *Eczema, 27 patients*—occurred when an individual felt that he was being interfered with or prevented from doing something and could think of no way to deal with the frustration. Typical statements included: "I want to make my mother understand, but I can't." "I take it out on myself."

3. *Cold and moist hands, 10 patients*—occurred when an individual felt that he should undertake some kind of activity, even though he might not know precisely what to do. "I just had to be doing something."

4. *Vasomotor rhinitis (runny nose), 12 patients*—occurred when an individual was facing a situation he couldn't do anything about. He wished that it would go away or that somebody else would take over the responsibility. The mucous membrane began to hypersecrete to wash out the foreign substance and get rid of it. "I wanted to blot it all out. I wanted to build a wall between me and him." "I wanted to go to bed and pull the sheets over my head."

5. *Asthma, 7 patients*—occurred in association with attitudes exactly like those associated with a runny nose. "I couldn't face it." "I wanted them to go away."

6. *Diarrhea, 27 patients*—occurred when an individual wanted to be done with a situation or to have it over with, or to get rid of something or somebody. "I wanted to crawl into a hole until it was all done." "I wanted to erase it from my life forever."

7. *Constipation, 17 patients*—occurred when an individual was grimly determined to carry on even when faced with a problem he could not solve. "I have to keep on with this, but I don't like it." "I'll stick with it although nothing good will come of it."

8. *Nausea and vomiting, 11 patients*—occurred when an individual was thinking of something he wished had never happened. He was preoccupied with the mistake he had made rather than with what he should have done instead. "I wish it never would have happened." "I made a mistake."

9. *Duodenal ulcer, 9 patients*—occurred when an individual was seeking revenge. He wished to injure the person or thing that had injured him. "I wanted to get back at him." "He hurt me so I wanted to hurt him." "This is just eating me up inside."

10. *Arterial hypertension, 7 patients*—occurred when an individual felt that he must be constantly prepared to meet all possible threats. "Nobody is ever going to beat me. I'm ready for anything." "It was up to me to take care of all the worries."

11. *Lower back pain, 11 patients*—occurred when an individual wanted to carry out some action involving movement of the entire body. The activity these patients were most commonly thinking about was walking or running away from a situation. "I just wanted to walk out of the house." "I wanted to run away."

12. *Migraine headache, 14 patients*—occurred when an individual had been making an intense effort to carry out a definite planned program or to achieve some definite objective. The headache occurred when the effort had ceased, no matter whether the activity had been associated with

> success or failure. “I had to get it done.” “I had a million things to do before lunch.” “I was trying to get all these things accomplished.”

### KINESIS

Kinesis is the study of body movement. Body movement is made possible through the use of muscles that are stimulated by nerves. Nerves are basically transporters of impulses. Impulses find their source in the control center called the brain. The thought process in the brain stimulates the nerve impulses. We have both voluntary impulses (like smiling at a friend and frowning at an enemy) and involuntary impulses that keep our heart pumping and our breathing continuous.

Kinesis not only studies the motion itself but also the relationship of the motion to the thinking process. You really cannot separate the mind and the body. We are our bodies mentally, emotionally, and physically.

Psychologist Wilhelm Reich believed that what happens in the mind is reflected in the body. He believed that chronic muscular tension and contraction produces rigidity. He called this constant contraction “muscular armor.” He also believed that this “armoring” was connected to an individual’s character and how he handled difficult situations.

One of Reich’s students, Dr. Alexander Lowen, expanded on this theory and developed a therapy called *Bioenergetics.* This particular approach focuses on the physical symptoms of “armoring” or pain spots. Lowen believed that you could reduce the armoring through massage, special exercises, and pressure on the muscles. That would, in turn, help the individual deal more effectively with their psychological problems.

It is believed that movement of various muscle groups helps to bleed off or release the armoring created by tension. This type of therapy has been helpful with tension headaches. Are you aware of any areas of your back, neck, jaw, or forehead that have been in a state of tension for a long period of time?

Closely aligned to Bioenergetics is *Rolfing*. This technique for releasing tension was developed by Ida P. Rolf, an organic chemist. It involves deep tissue massage. It usually involves ten one-hour sessions.

The deep tissue massage is temporarily a very painful process. A great deal of pressure is applied with the purpose of releasing tension and realigning the body. Many who have utilized Rolfing Therapy testify to feeling more natural and relaxed.

*Chiropractic* treatments utilize adjustments to the back, neck, hips, legs, and feet. When the back is misaligned (out of place), it causes pressure on nerves, which in turn cause muscles to spasm. It has been indicated that small shifts in the vertebrae (spinal subluxations) can cause mild to very sharp pain. This pain in specific locations can be relieved by physical manipulation being applied on those particular spots or general areas that are connected in a sort of rippling effect.

Chiropractic adjustments can many times instantly eliminate headache pain. This is especially true if an individual has been involved in an accident that has caused misalignment.

Although many people look down on chiropractic therapy, thousands of people will attest to finding relief from pain. I personally have experienced relief through chiropractic treatments from accidents and sports-related injuries. Many of the people that I have counseled have found chiropractic to be very beneficial. The father of medicine, Hippocrates, said, "In case of illness, look to the spine first."

*Feldenkrais exercises* have been helpful in reducing all sorts of pain, including headaches. These exercises were developed by Moshe Feldenkrais, a doctor in physics and the director of the Feldenkrais Institute in Tel Aviv.

Dr. Feldenkrais devised a system to affect neuromotor action and reconditioning. He believed that all body action involved movement, sensation, feeling, and thought. He also believed that we develop habits of physical response to common and difficult situations in life. How we carry ourselves when we walk, how we stand, how we hold our head, stomach, or hands, and how we express ourselves through our faces are all part of a "muscle and nerve memory system." They are part of our self-image.

To illustrate this, take a moment and try this exercise. Fold your arms across your chest. Next, unfold them and refold them the opposite way across your chest. Does it feel comfortable or uncomfortable? Is it easy to do this, or did you have a moment of difficulty where you had to think about what you were doing? Now, do the same type of thing with your hands. Interlace your fingers (clasp your hands) as you normally would do. Next, unlace them and lace them again the opposite way. Does it feel comfortable?

The reason one way feels comfortable and the other doesn't is because of "muscle and nerve memory." Dr. Feldenkrais suggests that we not only have a muscle and nerve memory for physical things but also for how we handle intellectual and emotional things in life. He believed that to change thinking processes we have to become aware of what is happening in our body. This awareness can be approached through muscle movement.

For example, you may not be aware of how you are breathing while you are reading this. But if I ask you to take a deep breath several times in a row (muscle movement), you suddenly become aware of your habit pattern of breathing. Were you breathing deep or shallow before I asked you to take a breath?

To approach the relief of headaches, we must first become aware of what is happening physically. It is then that we can do something (action) to change what is causing the pain. The awareness-action system is the way to approach change.

## CONSCIOUSNESS VS. AWARENESS

There is a distinct difference between consciousness and awareness. I can be conscious that I park my car in a lot and go shopping. I can return from shopping and be conscious that I am going back to my car. We all have done this. Now if I were to ask you how many cars you walked past in going to the store, that would be awareness. If I asked you the different colors of the cars you passed walking back from shopping to your car—that would be awareness. There is a difference.

You can be conscious that you have a headache. But you may not be aware of what has brought about the headache. This is what this whole book is about—making you aware of what is happening. It is only then that change can take place. This is true of headaches and most emotional issues we face in life.

*Massage* of muscles has been used throughout the ages to help bring about relaxation of the body. The massaging of the neck, shoulders, and back is beneficial in relieving headaches. When you massage the muscles of a friend or loved one, you will often hear comments like, "I'll give you an hour to stop that." Why? Because it feels so good.

There is a multimillion-dollar sales market that produces nothing but massage items. There are foot massagers, back massagers, table massagers, and chair massagers. They go fast and slow. They come with and without heat attachments. I have three different types in my own home.

Mechanical massagers are purchased because most people cannot afford to get a professional massage every time they would like one. Mechanical massagers are popular because your friend or loved one gets tired of giving you a massage. It involves hard work, and their hands and arms get tired.

*Therapeutic touch* can be an important help in relieving headaches. Ashley Montagu wrote a 512-page book titled *Touching: The Human Significance of the Skin*. In his book, he lists study after study that details the therapeutic importance of touching. He illustrates how newborn babies will die without touch. Young people need touching. People going through crisis and tragedy need to be touched. Older people need touching. Just go to any senior citizen home and give hugs to people, and you will see the positive response.

The act of touching lets the other person know that you care. It helps him to realize that he is not alone. It gives support and hope. A classic example is what happens when a small child gets hurt. The parent scoops the child into his or her arms and kisses away the pain. What is the magic that happens? Even though there may be an abrasion, wound, or bump, the crying dies away. Comfort is received. The area may still be sore, but there is relief from pain because of the touch and caring of another person.

A good medical example of this is mentioned in *Free Yourself From Pain* by Dr. David E. Bresler, director of the UCLA Pain Control Unit. He talks about Dr. Robert Swearingen, an orthopedic surgeon at the University of Colorado School of Medicine. Dr. Swearingen treats hundreds of serious injuries from the Colorado ski slopes. He has taught the ski patrol rescuers to take off their gloves and place one hand on the neck of the injured person and gently stroke the face with the other hand, saying, "Everything's going to be OK. You've hurt yourself, but we're here to take care of you now. Just relax and take it easy, and you're going to be fine." The very act of skin-to-skin touching and the soft gentle voice has worked wonders in relaxing injured people.

He goes on to say that when Dr. Swearingen has to treat a dislocated shoulder (which can be extremely painful), he does not anesthetize the person. He gently touches the shoulder and helps the person to breathe deep and relax. "Try and relax this muscle... ah, that's better... let it relax completely... very good... let yourself relax as much as you ever have before." He goes on to say, "You might feel a little pop as your shoulder comes back in, but because these muscles are completely relaxed, it won't hurt." And it doesn't.[4]

Studies have found that in some cases, the onset of asthma has a relationship to the lack of touching. Babies who are touched gain more weight than babies who are not touched. Touch can slow heartbeat and blood pressure. Anxiety levels can be reduced by touching. The elderly and those who are sick become calm and relaxed by petting animals. Children with psychological problems have a reduction in anxiety through touch. Touching is more common in Latin American countries than in the United States and England.

We can exercise the same therapeutic touch when it comes to headaches. We can help others to relax. We can let them know we are there and that we care. We can talk with gentle words and help them to breathe deeply. We can gently stroke their forehead, top of their head, and the back of their head and neck. You will be amazed at the benefits both parties receive from touching in a caring manner.

## BIOFEEDBACK

Biofeedback is a technique for helping individuals become aware of tension in their body. It provides objective information about muscle activity, body temperature, and brain waves.

The feedback of what is happening in the body is accomplished by three methods. The first involves placing electrodes on various places of the body. The electrodes identify muscle activity (tension) and convey that information to a machine. The machine will register the levels of muscle activity in two ways. One is to have a visual meter indicating the degree of muscle activity. The other is to have an audible signal (a noise) that raises and lowers according to the degree of muscle activity. This is called EMG—electromyographic biofeedback.

The individual who is hooked up to the biofeedback machine is then taught methods of relaxation. As the person begins to relax various muscle areas in his or her body, the visual tension meter will go down and the auditory sound will decrease. The person can learn to control blood pressure, muscle tension, skin temperature in the hands, and even movement in the digestive system.

After a number of training sessions on the biofeedback machine, individuals can then apply the same relaxation techniques when they are not on the machine. At the Diamond Health Clinic in

Chicago, one study indicated that 68 percent of those who were taught biofeedback relaxation methods were able to reduce the frequency and duration of their headaches following the training.[5]

Biofeedback is a safe method to make the invisible (muscle tension) visible and audible. Headache sufferers can learn to relax and calm the muscles of the forehead, neck, and back. They also learn the importance of breathing correctly.

The second method of recording biofeedback involves the use of thermometers to register the temperature of the hands. It is called *thermal feedback*. Headache sufferers have a tendency to have cold hands. This is an indication of the flow of adrenaline in the body, which is causing a decrease of blood flow to the hands. Normal hand temperature is in the 90–96 degree area. Those who are experiencing adrenaline flow, muscle tension, and headaches can have their hand temperature drop into the low-70s degree area. The tension in the body gives itself away by the presence of cold hands unless it is just plain cold outside.

For a moment, test and see if your hands are cold or warm. Place both of your palms on each side of your face. Do your hands feel warm or cool? If your face feels warm, then your hands are cooler than your face. Do the back of your hands feel warm or cool?

Headache sufferers are then taught the same relaxation methods as those using the EMG machines. They learn how to increase the temperature of their hands, which helps to reduce their headache severity and frequency. Although reduction in headaches can be accomplished this way, the process of how it works is not fully understood.

We are not talking about running your hands under hot water—although that can help to some degree. What we are suggesting is warming your hands from the inside out.

This amazing process can be accomplished by finding a quiet spot and sitting or lying down. The object is to relax your body and mentally concentrate on warming your hands.

Sometimes it is helpful to have soft music playing in the background to aid in relaxation. It is also helpful to begin to think about a favorite place you like to go—like the beach, mountains, or some calming spot you like to retreat to. Imagine that you are in that location and are feeling the warmth of the sun on your body. You imagine how pleasant it feels and how it begins to warm you. Begin to concentrate on the sun warming your hands. "I can feel my hands becoming warmer and warmer."

At the same time that you are concentrating on warming your hands, begin to breathe deeply. Slowly draw in a breath to the count of six...hold your breath for the count of six...slowly let out your breath to the count of six.

It is ideal to attempt to do this twice a day if you can. Try and set aside ten to twenty minutes for the exercise. If you tape a thermometer to your finger or hold one of the new battery-operated thermometers, you can actually begin to see your cold hands begin to become warmer. This indicates that your body is beginning to relax and muscle tension is reducing, which in turn helps to reduce muscle tension headaches.

Cold hands can also be the result of a disease called Raynaud's syndrome. It is the result of poor circulation. Those with diabetes could also be experiencing cold hands.

The third method is to use an EEG—electroencephalograph machine. Electrodes are placed on the head to monitor brain waves. Again, the individual is taught relaxation techniques, as with the other two methods.

After a number of training sessions with any of the three biofeedback methods, the individual can learn to raise their hand temperature, control muscle tension, and help reduce headaches. These techniques can be reinforced through daily practice and during stressful situations.

## EXERCISE, AEROBIC AND ANAEROBIC

Our bodies were designed for movement. Our muscles need to be exercised to remain healthy and flexible. Physical activity helps to bleed off stress and muscle tension that lead to headaches. Except for extreme exertion or a quick sudden movement, rarely do people experience headaches when exercising. Exercise helps to reduce the frequency and duration of headaches.

When people experience chronic pain, a sedentary lifestyle retards the healing process. Movement and physical activity are the natural response to stress. Movement decreases the muscle cramping and stiffness. Muscles that do not move, or exercise, begin to lose their strength, and atrophy sets in.

Aerobic exercise relies on oxygen. Activities that demand more oxygen include walking, jogging, bicycling, swimming, tennis, dancing, racquetball, and skipping rope. It is best that these physical exercises last at least twenty to thirty minutes and are done three to four times a week.

Anaerobic exercises rely more on quick, short-term bursts of energy. They include fast movements for a short period like jumping, throwing, or weight lifting. Deep relaxation usually follows aerobic and anaerobic exercise about ninety minutes after the workout session. Often exercise releases endorphins, which help the body to feel good.

For a number of years I was involved with karate. The exercises are very strenuous and require both anaerobic and aerobic involvement. I could come to the karate class tired, stressed out, and emotionally drained from work. After the workout I would leave feeling more relaxed, energetic, and inwardly calm.

## ACTIVITY ASSESSMENT TEST

Listed below are activities that are common for a twenty-four hour period. You may engage in an activity that is not listed. Try and approximate that activity with one similar to those listed. Multiply the weighted score for the activity by the time you spend in that activity. Fifteen minutes spent would equal .25;

thirty minutes spent would equal .50; forty-five minutes spent would equal .75; and one hour spent would equal 1.0 times the weighted score. When completed, total the points. This will give you your daily activity score.[6]

| ACTIVITY ASSESSMENT TEST | | | |
|---|---|---|---|
| *How many hours per day do you spend…?* | | | |
| **ACTIVITY** | **HOURS** | **POINTS PER HOUR** | **TOTAL POINTS** |
| Sleeping | | 0.85 | |
| Sitting: Riding/driving | | 1.5 | |
| Sitting: Study/desk work | | 1.5 | |
| Sitting: Meals | | 1.5 | |
| Sitting: Watching TV | | 1.5 | |
| Sitting: Reading | | 1.5 | |
| Sitting: Other | | 1.5 | |
| Standing | | 2.0 | |
| Standing: Dressing | | 2.0 | |
| Standing: Showering | | 2.0 | |
| Standing: Other | | 2.0 | |
| Walking: Slow walk | | 3.0 | |

**ACTIVITY ASSESSMENT TEST**

*How many hours per day do you spend . . . ?*

| ACTIVITY | HOURS | POINTS PER HOUR | TOTAL POINTS |
|---|---|---|---|
| Walking: Moderate speed | | 4.0 | |
| Walking: Very fast walk | | 5.0 | |
| Housework, light physical work | | 3.0 | |
| Rapid calisthenics | | 4.0 | |
| Slow run (jog) | | 6.0 | |
| Fast run | | 7.0 | |
| Racket sports | | 8.0 | |
| Competitive sports | | 9.0–10.0 | |
| Stair climbing | | 8.0 | |
| TOTAL HOURS INVOLVED | 24 | TOTAL POINTS | |

Do you have an exercise outlet for stress buildup? ☐ Yes ☐ No

Do you use it? ☐ Yes ☐ No

Do you exercise regularly for its preventive rewards? ☐ Yes ☐ No

Have you discovered the psychological and emotional benefits of exercise? ☐ Yes ☐ No

Do you want to begin a regular program of exercise? ☐ Yes ☐ No

Scores of 40 or below—You are a very sedentary person.
Stores of 55 or more—You are probably enjoying the benefits of physical activity.

Dr. Robert S. Ivker, in his book *Headache Survival,* recounts a very interesting study.

> A seven-year study conducted by the University of Minnesota School of Public Health tracked the physical activity levels of over 40,000 women, all of whom were postmenopausal and ranged in age from fifty-five to sixty-nine. The results showed that women who exercised at least four times a week at high intensity had up to a 30-percent lowered risk of early death compared to women in the same age group who were sedentary.[7]

If, for various reasons, you cannot presently be involved in a heavy exercise program—you can exercise in other ways. But before beginning any exercise program, consult your family physician. When you go shopping, park your car farther away from the building rather than closer. Number one, you will be guaranteed a parking place, and number two, you will get extra exercise from walking a distance. Instead of using an elevator, walk up and down the stairs. Spend part of your lunch hour going for a walk around the block or around your building. Walk backwards for short distances. If you live close to a store, walk rather than drive. Take a brisk walk in the evening. A good walk will do wonders for emotional turmoil, stress from work, depression, and headaches. Do your own yard work rather than hiring someone to do it for you. Attempt to break out of the sedentary lifestyle.

### HELPFUL DESK EXERCISES

Finding time to exercise, especially for those who work more than sixty hours a week, is not always easy. At times you may feel as if you are chained to your desk. If you are one of those who say, "I just can't afford to take a fifteen-minute break; I've got too many deadlines," now you have no excuse because you can do the following exercises and *still* be chained to your desk.

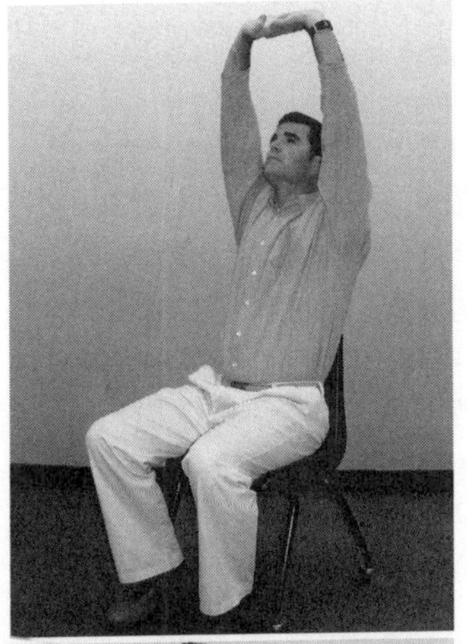

*Reach for the sky*

- Take a slow deep breath to the count of five.
- Raise your hands over your head at the same time; hold for five seconds.
- Slowly lower arms and breathe out; let shoulders sag.
- Repeat exercise seven times.

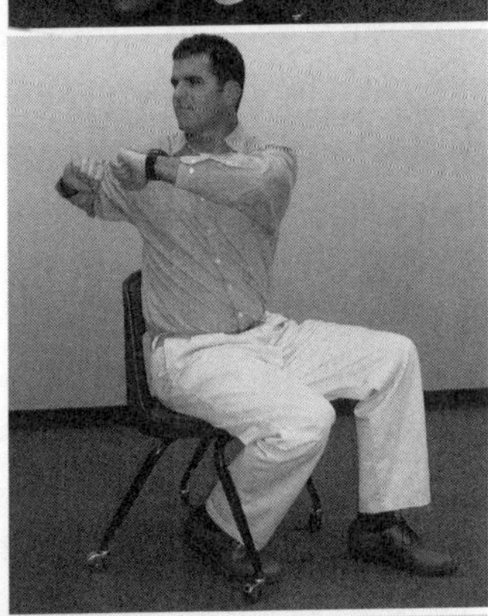

*Do the twist*

- Raise elbows to shoulder level.
- Twist to right and to the left as far as you can at a medium speed.
- Repeat the twisting a dozen times.
- Do not hold your breath while twisting from side to side.

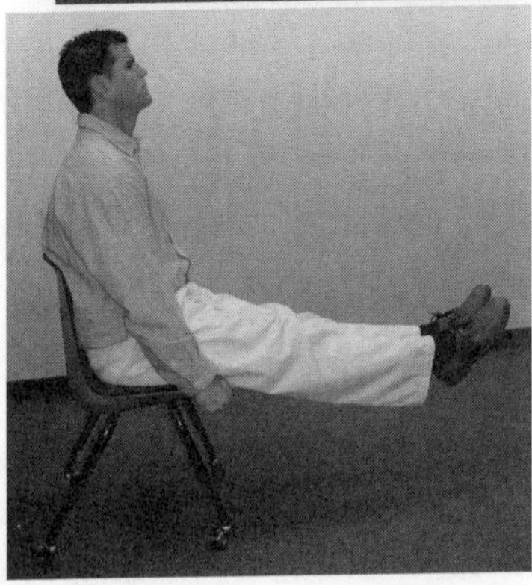

*Leg kicks*

- Hold on to chair.
- Raise feet off floor a couple of inches.
- Keep upper leg straight, and kick lower leg out straight in front.
- Relax and let lower leg swing back.
- Repeat, kicking legs forward twenty times.

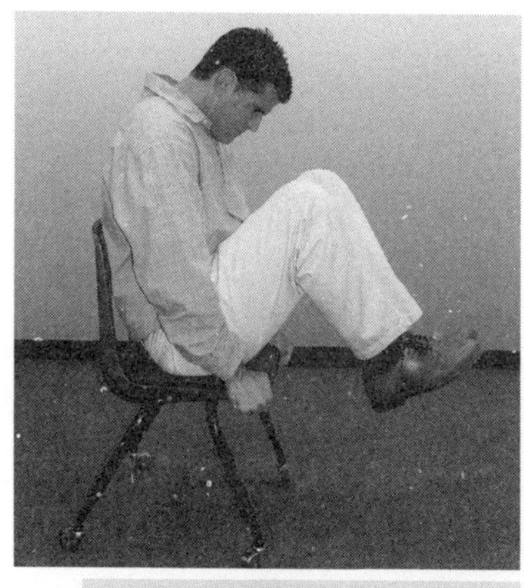

*Chair crunch*

- Hold on to chair.
- Draw legs up and bend upper body forward at the same time.
- Breathe out as you draw legs up; breathe in, then breathe out as legs return to the floor.
- Repeat exercise at least twelve times.

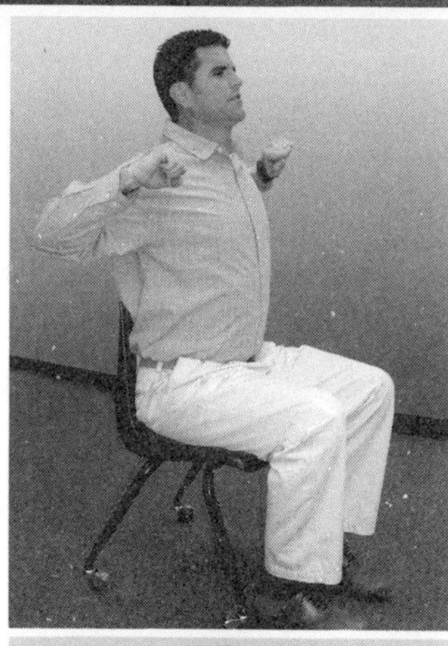

*Row your boat*

- Sit up straight with feet flat on floor.
- Sit forward, touching your hands to your feet.
- Sit back up, pulling elbows back in a rowing fashion—hold for a few seconds.
- Repeat exercise twenty times—exhale bending forward.

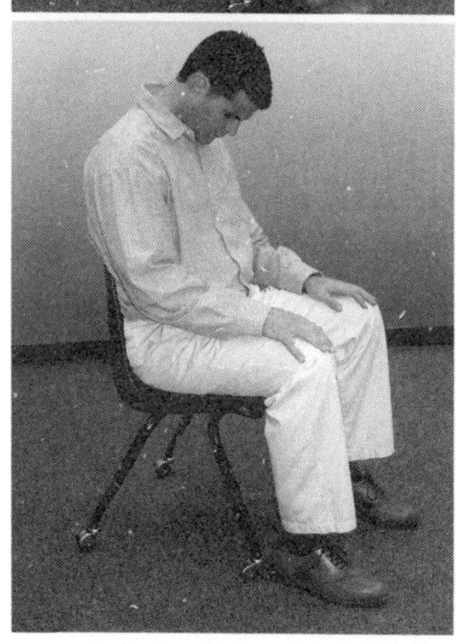

*Head rolls*

- Sit with hands on knees—shoulders relaxed.
- Bend head forward, and slowly make ten large circles to the right.
- Then slowly make ten large circles to the left.
- Keep motion slow and relaxed.

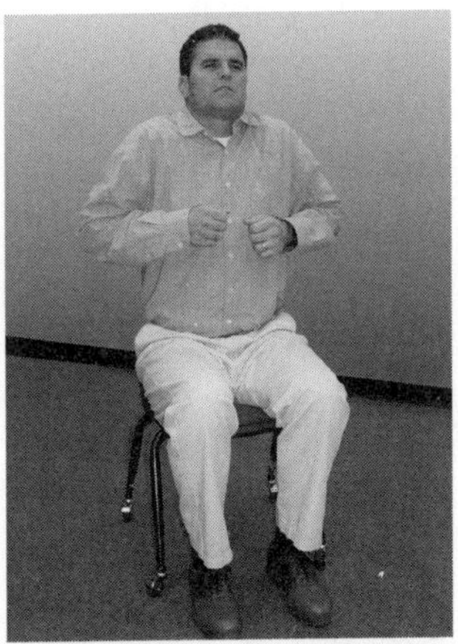

*Who me? shrugs*

- Sit up straight.
- Slowly raise your hands, and shrug shoulders up—hold five seconds.
- Slowly relax (breathing out and counting to five) while dropping hands to lap.
- Repeat exercise at least twelve times.

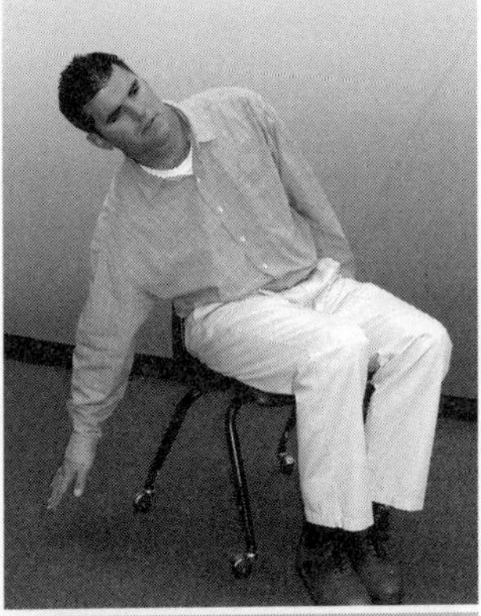

*Touch the floor*

- Sit up straight with bottom touching back of chair—arms hanging at sides.
- Slowly reach down to side (as far as you can) and touch the floor.
- Repeat exercise on both sides twelve times.

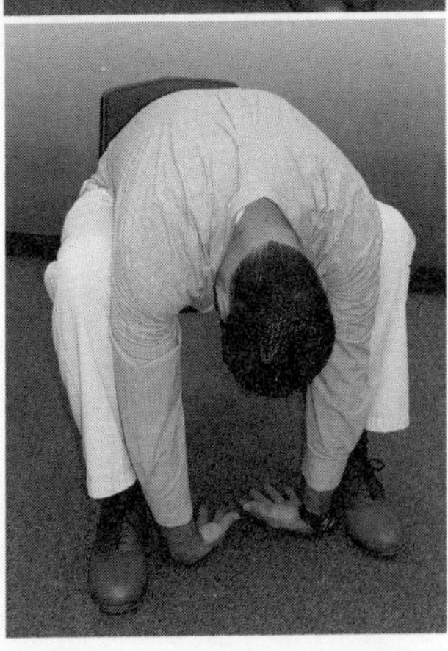

*Palms down*

- Sit back in your chair—feet about twelve inches apart.
- Bend forward and allow your palms to rest on the floor.
- Relax head, neck, and back—remain down for count of fifteen.
- Sit up; repeat exercise seven times.

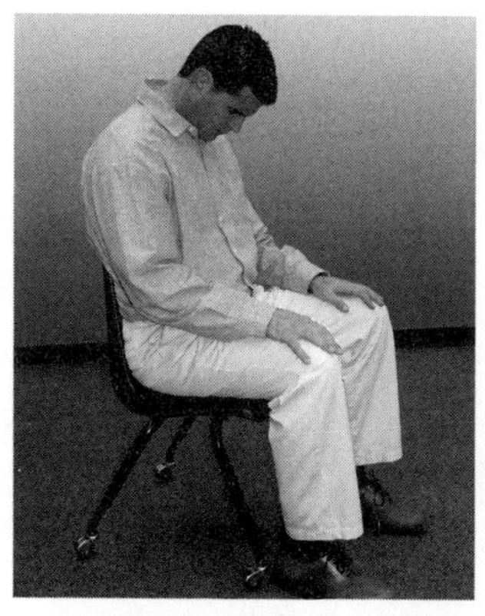

*Head drop*

- Sit with bottom and back against chair.
- Allow head to drop forward; feel neck and back muscles relaxing.
- Keep relaxing muscles—head seems to drop more and more.
- After thirty seconds, raise up and repeat exercise three times.

## PRESSURE

Applying pressure to the head can help to relieve some headaches. This can be accomplished by placing the palm of one hand to the forehead and the palm of the other hand to the back of the head. Apply as much pressure as you can—and hold it for as long as you can. Repeat this exercise about six times. Also, place the fingers and palms of your hands to the top of your head and press down as hard as you can for as long as you can. Repeat this action about six times.

Some people have found it helpful to wrap a belt around their head and squeeze it as tight as they can. This applies a uniform pressure around the entire head at the same time. After a period of time, the pressure is released. This is repeated about six times in a row or until relief is achieved.

*Hot and cold*

Many people achieve headache relief by applying cold packs or hot packs to their foreheads. Cold packs are especially helpful when there are headaches from fevers or the individual has a migraine headache. A cold pack in a darkened room while lying down is very soothing. Wrap an ice pack in a cloth to protect your skin from direct contact. Do not keep ice directly on the skin for long periods. Cold showers or a cold swim can be stimulating and invigorating.

Hot baths, steam rooms, and saunas bring about the relaxation of muscles that result in headaches from tension and anxiety. The breathing of moist air is also beneficial.

*Sleep and fatigue*

If you are having headaches, take a good look at your sleep pattern. The continued lack of sleep and the fatigue that comes from it can trigger headaches. What time do you go to bed? How many hours of sleep per night do you get?

The best sleep is achieved from 9:30 p.m. to 2:00 a.m. A comfortable mattress helps to make sleep more beneficial. A good pillow that eliminates cervical neck problems is essential. Making an effort to go to bed at the same time also helps the body to establish a good sleep routine.

Physical exercise before going to bed or using relaxation techniques can also help you get a good night's sleep. A good walk in the evening after dinner is a starting point. Most health professionals recommend you exercise at least four hours *before* bedtime and avoid strenuous exercise right before sleep.

Try moving your clock away from your view from the bed. This will help you not to be counting minutes. As long as the clock is within eyesight, it is easy to keep looking at the clock to see how long you have been awake.

Most people lead busy lives with hectic schedules, so it is easy for the mind to think about all the things to be accomplished the next day. We lie awake thinking about them and worrying that we will forget something that needs to be done. If that's you, then keep a pad and a pen next to your bed. When the thoughts come, write them down. This way, you can relax and go to sleep because you have a list written.

If for some reason you still cannot go to sleep, you might be wise to get up. Nothing is worse than tossing and turning and wasting time. Otherwise you might wake up tired, angry, or frustrated. You might find it helpful to go to work and accomplish some household task, business responsibility, exercise, or catch up on reading. Why? Because you are going to be awake anyway. Why not at least accomplish some task that needs to be done? In this way, at least something positive has been done rather than throwing away the precious time.

## STRETCHING EXERCISES

Stretching exercises can be used to help relieve headaches that are caused by tension and stress. These exercises will help to develop muscle tone and circulation of the blood, and they will help to eliminate stiffness and soreness.

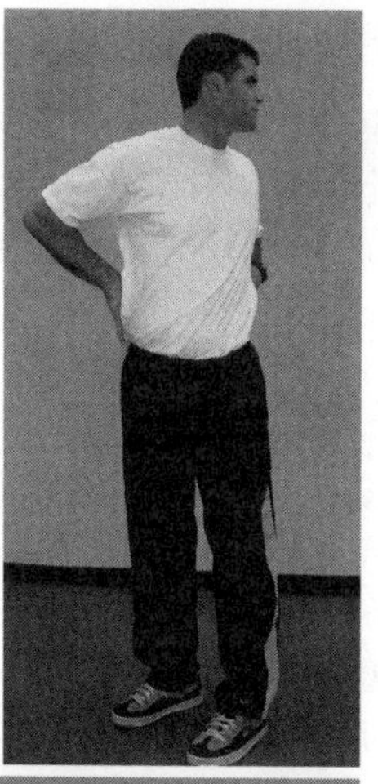

*Torso twist*

- Stand up with your feet shoulder-width apart.
- Put your arms behind your back.
- Twist to right and left while exhaling and inhaling.
- Repeat exercise at least twelve times in each direction.

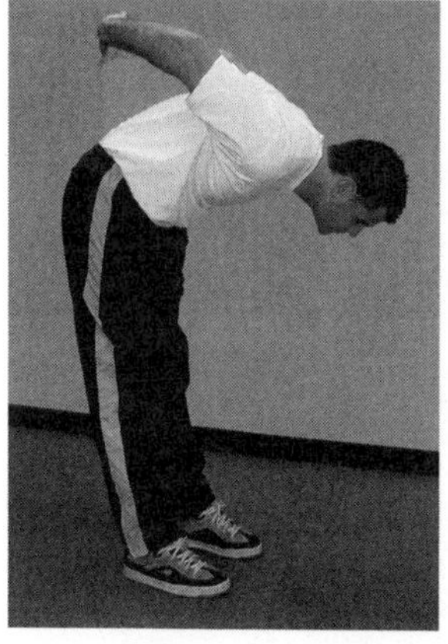

*Floor stretch*

- Stand with feet together.
- Lock hands together behind back and raise them up as you bend your body forward, breathing in and out; hold for five seconds.
- Alternate with back bend.

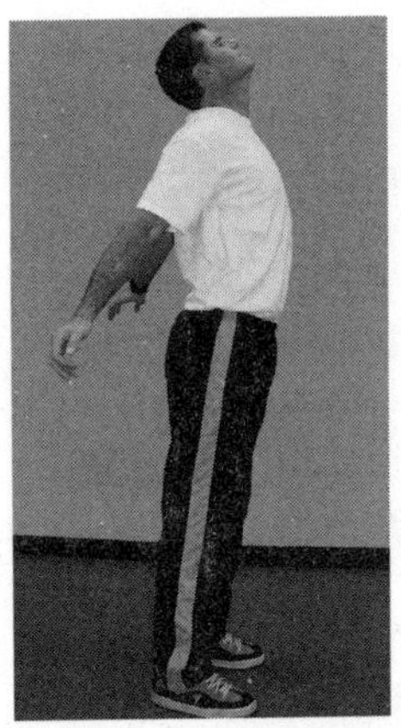

*Back bend*

- Stand with feet together.
- Arch backwards after floor stretch, letting your hands drop. Don't get off balance.
- Hold for five seconds.
- Alternate floor stretch and back bend at least twelve times.

To test your flexibility, you might experiment with this exercise. Place a 12- to 16-inch box on the floor. Next, get a yardstick and let the first 12 inches hang over the box. Sit on the floor with your legs together and straight out in front of you. The bottoms of your feet should be flat against the box.

Now, bend forward with your hands over the yardstick. Reach as far as you can and measure how many inches it is. Do this exercise three times. Note what your best stretching reach is. Excellent flexibility will be from 20 to 21 inches. Very good flexibility will be from 17 to 19 inches. Good flexibility will be from 15 to 16 inches. Fair flexibility will be from 10 to 14 inches. Low flexibility will be from 7 to 9 inches. Poor flexibility will be anything less than 6 inches.

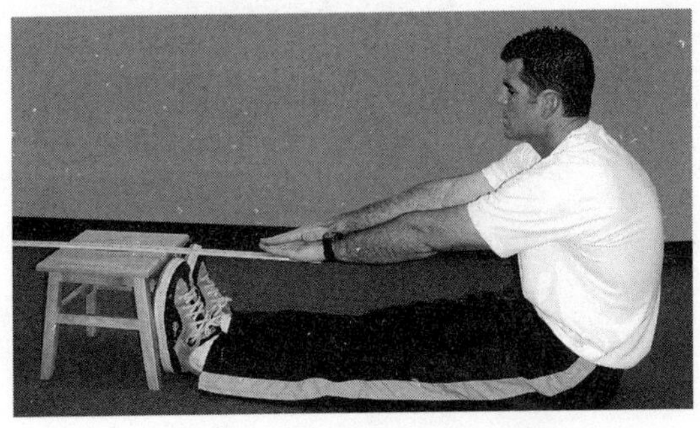

## TENS

Headache relief can be found by utilizing an electrical device called *TENS.* The acronym TENS stands for "Transcutaneous Electrical Nerve Stimulator." This is a low-voltage portable unit that looks similar to a transistor radio or a beeper. It generates a pulsating electrical impulse to small electrodes taped to the skin. The electrodes are usually placed on the neck, shoulders, or back.

The nerve stimulator interrupts normal nerve impulses that send pain messages. The individual wearing the TENS unit can control (turn on and off) the stimulation as needed. This helps to give independence and freedom from headache pain. TENS does not work for all headaches. However, over 50 percent of the people using these units testify to positive results. TENS units must be prescribed by a physician.

Closely related to the TENS units are the SEA stimulators. *SEA* stands for "Synaptic Electronic Activation." These are high-frequency electrical generators that deliver stimulation on a much higher level of frequency. The impulses travel along the nerve pathway to the nerve synapse and assist in pain relief. This is caused by helping to modify the neurotransmitters, which release the endorphins, serotonin, and epinephrine, and can last up to twenty-four hours. The SEA stimulator has controls that allow the individual to control the intensity of the impulses sent to the nerves.[8]

Over the years, doctors and researchers have discovered the importance of physical strategies for health. Simple things like stretching, breathing, and proper sleep are effective methods for dealing with headaches. Alignment, posture, and stimulating acupressure points been have proven to reduce the pain associated with headaches. But do not stop at physical methods in exploring headache pain reduction. It is also important to understand the effects of diet and medicine on the human body.

CHAPTER 11

# Diet and Medical Strategies for Headache Relief

*He who has health has hope, and he who has hope has everything.*[1]

Many people are not aware of the close tie between what they put into their bodies and the headaches they experience. They do not realize that various foods and beverages can cause their headache pain. As a result, they continue to experience headaches that could otherwise be controlled.

## ALCOHOL

Many headaches are brought on by or made worse by alcohol. Alcohol is what is called a *vasodilator.* It causes the blood vessels to dilate, or open up. This stretching of the fine muscles of the blood vessels provokes headaches. It can produce what is called the "hangover" headache.

Alcohol is created by a fermentation process that produces tyramine, histamine, acetaldehyde, and acetate. Many people are allergic to sulfites contained in alcohol. Red wine has a good portion of tyramine in it. Some alcohol contains additives like esters, acids, and tannins, which irritate some people.

Those who experience headaches while drinking wine or other forms of alcohol would be wise to reduce their intake or completely eliminate it from their diet.

It is also good to remember that vinegars also go through a fermentation process. People who may not be drinking alcohol may still ingest tyramine. Eating products like ketchup, mustard, mayonnaise, and pickled products that use vinegar might be the cause of your headaches because of the tyramine found in vinegar.

## ALLERGIES

Allergies affect a large portion of people in the United States. An allergy is the body's negative reaction to a food, animal, or chemical. The histamine levels in the body increase and can produce reactions of stomach pain, nausea, cramps, vomiting, diarrhea, rash, swelling, tearing of eyes, nasal congestion, headaches, closing of airways, and life-threatening anaphylaxis. Listed below are foods that can cause headaches or produce allergies in some people.

| ALLERGY-PRODUCING AND HEADACHE-CAUSING FOODS | | | |
|---|---|---|---|
| Accent seasoning | Alcohol | Anchovies | Aspartame (NutraSweet, Equal) |
| Avocados | Bacon | Bagels | Baking mixes |
| Bananas | Beef jerky | Bologna | Bouillon cubes |
| Bread with yeast | Bread stuffing | Breaded foods | Broad beans |
| Buttermilk | Cane sugar | Canned ham | Canned meats |
| Caviar | Cheese | Cheese dips | Chicken dogs |
| Chocolate | Citrus fruits | Clam chowder | Coffee |
| Colas | Cold foods | Cole slaw | Corn chips |
| Corned beef | Croutons | Dates | Doughnuts |
| Eggplant | Eggs | Fatty foods | Figs (canned) |
| Frozen dinners | Frozen pizza | Garbanzo beans | Gelatins |
| Hamburger Helper | Herring | Hot dogs | Instant gravies |

| ALLERGY-PRODUCING AND HEADACHE-CAUSING FOODS | | | |
|---|---|---|---|
| Ketchup | Lawry's Seasoning Salt | Lentils | Lima beans |
| Liverwurst | Low-calorie foods | Marinated food | Mayonnaise |
| Monosodium | MSG | Mushrooms | Mustard |
| Navy beans | Nuts | Onions | Organ meats |
| Oriental food | Packaged tenderizers | Papayas | Pea pods |
| Peanut butter | Pepperoni | Peppers | Pineapple |
| Pinto beans | Pizza dough | Plums | Pot pies |
| Potato chips | Potatoes | Processed cheeses | Processed meats |
| Raisins | Raspberries | Raw garlic | Red plums |
| Relishes | Saccharin (Sweet'n Low) | Salad dressings | Salami |
| Salt substitutes | Sauerkraut | Sausage | Seasonings |
| Self-basting turkeys | Sesame seeds | Smoked fish | Soft pretzels |
| Soups | Sour cream | Soy sauce | Spinach |
| String beans | Sunflower seeds | Tea | Tomatoes |
| Turkey dogs | Veggie burgers | Vinegars | Wheat |
| Wines | Yeast | Yogurt | |

After looking over this list, you might become a bit depressed. You may ask, "What am I going to eat or drink in life?" The purpose of this list is not to say that you should *never* eat any of these foods. It is only to alert you to the fact that headaches can be produced from many sources.

If you suspect that you have an allergy, it is important that you go to your physician and be tested. The elimination of a food-producing allergen could help bring you to health.

If you suspect that one or more of these foods might be causing your headaches or making them worse, then eliminate them from your diet for a period of one month. During that month, be sure to keep a good headache diary that will note the decrease in frequency or duration of headaches. If there is no change, add that particular food back into your regular eating pattern. This may be a slow process of elimination, but you will save big dollars in doctor visits.

## FATS

There is a lot of talk about too much fat in the diet of Americans. Fats can increase cholesterol in the body. Cholesterol promotes platelet clustering. This, in turn, reduces the levels of serotonin in the bloodstream, which cause the blood vessels to dilate. The dilation of blood vessels can begin to produce the pain of headaches.

The bottom line is that we cannot eliminate all fat from our diets. Nor should we do so. We do need some fats. What we are talking about is reducing the intake of fats. Studies indicate that as fat levels decrease, so do the frequency and duration of headaches.

Another thought to keep in mind when eating fats is to drink plenty of water. Water inhibits and makes it more difficult for the body to digest fats. It is important to remind ourselves of the Food Pyramid recommended by the United States Department of Agriculture.

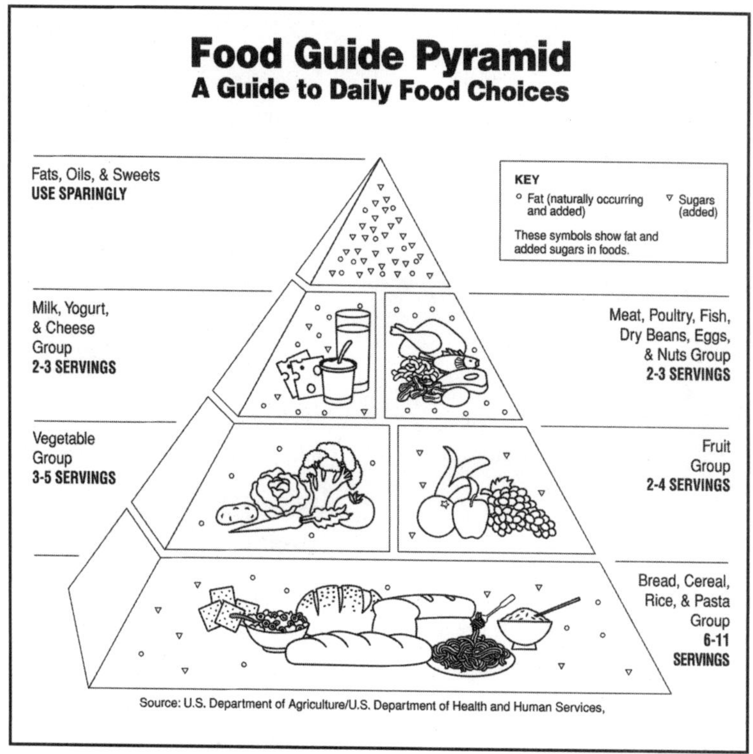


Notice that fats and sweets should be the smallest amounts of your daily intake. If you keep your fat intake to a minimum, it will not only help with headaches, but it will also keep you healthy.

## MEDICATIONS

Thus far in this chapter we have been talking about strategies and preventative treatments. Now we want to address medications. Medications do not prevent the *causes* of headaches. They are designed to treat the *result* of headaches. And, unfortunately in many cases, *medications themselves are the cause of headaches.* Listed below are some of the medications (drugs) that can have headache as a possible side effect:

| MEDICATIONS THAT CAN CAUSE HEADACHES | | | |
|---|---|---|---|
| Achromycin | Adalat | AeroBid | Allerest |
| Anacin | Aristocort | Bactrim | Brevicon |
| Cafergot | Capoten | Cibalith-S | Celestone |
| Comtrex | Contac | Cortef | Cortone |
| Cylert | Darvon | Decadron | Detrol |
| Delta-Cortef | Deltasone | Demerol | Demulen |
| Dexedrine | Didrex | Dilantin | Dilatrate-SR |
| Dilaudid | Dimetapp | Dristan | Enovid |
| Excedrin | Feldene | Fulvicin | Haldrone |
| Hytrin | Indocin | Intron A | Lithane |
| Lithobid | Lo/Ovral | Lopressor | Marplan |
| Minitran | Nardil | Nasacort | NegGram |
| Nitro-Bid | Nitrodisc | Nitro-Dur | Nitrogard |
| Nitrolingual | Nitrong | Nitrostat | Norinyl |
| Ortho-Novum | Ovcan | Ovral | Panmycin |
| Parnate | Percocet | Pondimin | Preludin |
| Prozac | Ritalin | Robitet | Sanorex |
| Septra | Sinarest | Sorbitrate | Sumycin |
| Tagamet | Tenormin | Tavist-D | Triphasil |
| Tylenol | Tylox | Vicodin | Voltaren |
| Zantac | | | |

For most people, when a headache comes, they want quick, immediate relief. This is, of course, very understandable. Their head hurts, and they don't like the feeling of pain and discomfort.

The most common and most usual course of action is to reach for a pain reducer. Over-the-counter drugs like aspirin, Excedrin, Anacin, Tylenol, and Aleve are very popular painkillers. They seem to provide a quick-fix relief.

Many of these pain medications contain caffeine. Caffeine has a tendency to constrict blood vessels and help reduce swelling. As the swelling goes down, the pain is reduced. The person feels better.

However, as the pain medication is absorbed and is passed out of the body, the swelling (headache) returns. Only this time, it swells even more, causing increased pain. The individual then again reaches for more pain medication, and the vicious cycle of "rebound headaches" begins. The headaches keep going and growing.

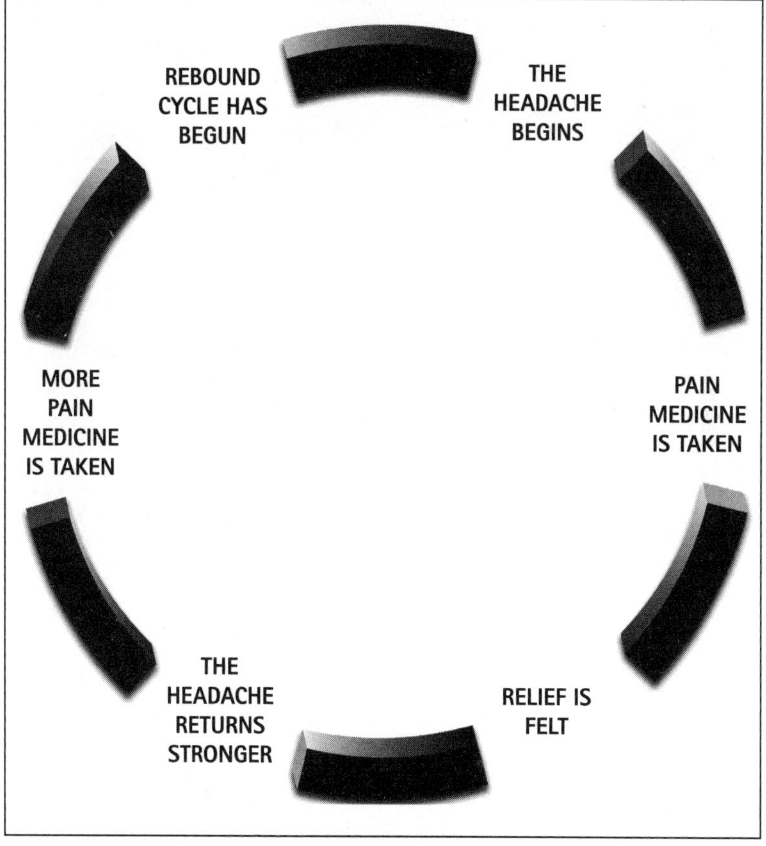


The vicious rebound cycle can begin to take the headache sufferer captive after weeks, months, or years. As the body begins to build up a resistance, the pain-killing feature wears off. The effect of the pain medicine decreases, and dependence on more and more painkillers is required. The individual is hooked. Are you hooked?

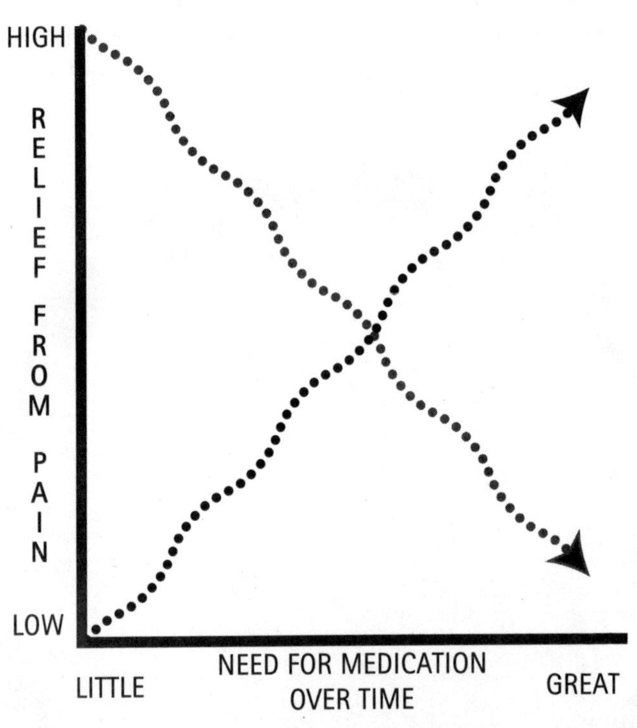


Unfortunately, many doctors contribute to the rebound cycle. They don't have the time and are too busy, they don't have the knowledge, or they don't take the energy to think about the long-term results of their actions. Millions of headache sufferers are in the same boat as the doctors. Instead of asking, "What medication should I take for headache relief?", headache sufferers should be asking, "How can I prevent headaches in the first place?" That is what this book is all about.

As a helpful hint, it is best to stop the rebound cycle before there is an attempt to work on preventative treatments. Continuing to take medication that may be causing headaches while trying to accomplish headache reduction is counterproductive.

You may ask, "Is it best to withdraw slowly or to do it all at once—cold turkey?" In most cases I think the "cold turkey" method will be more productive. By doing it slowly, there is always the temptation to drag out the process and never make a clean break.

As another helpful hint, you may experience withdrawals for about a week. In other words, your headache pain may increase for a short period. This is to be expected. Your body has gotten used to having it filled with painkillers. Don't be discouraged. The pain will diminish in most cases over a short period of time as the body's metabolism readjusts.

Is there ever justification for taking pain medication? Of course there is. Over-the-counter medications do bring temporary pain relief. However, it is best not to exceed them more than twice a month. Number one, they will begin to lose their effectiveness. Number two, it will begin to become costly. And last, you will come to depend on medication rather than learning to deal with the many causes for headaches on a preventive basis.

When it comes to prescription drugs, don't just accept them without questioning the doctor. Ask questions such as:

- "What will this drug do for me specifically?"
- "How long will I have to remain on this drug?'
- "What are the side effects of this drug?"
- "If I discontinue this drug, will I have withdrawal problems?"
- "Have you used this drug before? What have been the results?"
- "What will I do if I have problems taking this drug?"

If you find the doctor dancing around the questions, avoiding the questions, or giving you fuzzy answers—watch out! Don't be afraid to put him on the spot a little. It is your body. It is your money. The doctor works for you.

You will need to educate yourself in the area of drugs. Next time a drug is advertised on the TV, listen carefully. Listen to how quickly they rattle off the side effects of the drug. Ask yourself, *Would I want any one of those side effects to be in my life?* My guess is that you would say, "No!"

Have you ever wondered where most doctors get schooled in all the new drugs that are on the market? Do you think they are studying drug literature while you are sitting there in the lobby for great periods of time waiting for your appointment? Most doctors get their information from drug salesmen, leaflets, and samples left for them to try. They don't have the time or the energy to go to a lab and test the drugs themselves. They accept the information passed on to them by faith. So what else is new? We all do that.

I'm just attempting to encourage you to take a more active role in the management of your health care. No one cares about your health as much as *you* do. You are the only one who lives in your body. You are the best one to take care of it.

## VITAMINS AND MINERALS

Vitamins and minerals have been found to play an important role in the control of headaches.

Vitamins C and E contain beta carotene and help in the production of serotonin. Some studies indicate that riboflavin (vitamin $B_2$) assists in reducing migraines in up to 68 percent of those studied. Vitamin $B_6$ (pyridoxine) supports serotonin production. Vitamin $B_1$ (thiamine) aids in lowering blood fat. Magnesium contributes to vascular tone. Omega-3 facilitates the reduction of the frequency and intensity of migraines. Copper, zinc, and iron are involved in the metabolism of serotonin. Listed below are some of the sources of vitamins and minerals that contribute to the reduction of headaches.[2]

*Niacin*

- Brewer's yeast
- Green peas
- Potatoes
- Chicken
- Peanut butter
- Salmon

*Folic acid*

- Avocados
- Beets
- Broccoli
- Bulgur
- Okra
- Red beans
- Soybeans
- Wheat bread
- Bananas
- Brewer's yeast
- Brussels sprouts
- Kidney beans
- Orange juice
- Romaine lettuce
- Spinach
- Wheat germ

*Copper and zinc*

- Almonds
- Bananas
- Green peas
- Oysters
- Spinach
- Avocados
- Carrots
- Liver
- Potatoes
- Whole-wheat bread

*Iron*

- Apricots
- Lima beans
- Molasses
- Oysters
- Spinach
- Ground beef
- Liver
- Navy beans
- Raisins
- Split peas

*Magnesium and calcium*

- Avocados
- Beet greens
- Broccoli
- Cashews
- Bananas
- Brewer's yeast
- Brown rice
- Collard greens

- Kidney beans
- Navy beans
- Peanut butter
- Popcorn
- Rye flour
- Soy milk
- Tofu
- Whole-wheat bread
- Mustard greens
- Oranges
- Peanuts
- Pumpkin seeds
- Shrimp
- Spinach
- Wheat germ
- Yogurt

*Vitamin C*

- Bell peppers
- Broccoli
- Cantaloupe
- Kiwi fruit
- Papayas
- Black currants
- Brussels sprouts
- Grapefruit
- Oranges
- Strawberries

*Vitamin A*

- Apricots
- Cantaloupe
- Mangos
- Prunes
- Spinach
- Beet greens
- Carrots
- Persimmons
- Pumpkin
- Sweet potatoes

*Vitamin $B_6$*

- Avocados
- Bran cereal
- Corn flakes
- Oatmeal
- Rice bran
- Bananas
- Chickpeas
- Figs
- Potatoes
- Sweet potatoes

*Vitamin $B_3$*

- Bran cereals
- Buckwheat flour
- Halibut
- Peanut butter
- Rice
- Brewer's yeast
- Corn flakes
- Mushrooms
- Potatoes
- Tuna

*Vitamin $B_2$*

- Beet greens
- Brewer's yeast
- Milk
- Seaweed
- Spinach
- Bran cereals
- Corn flakes
- Mushrooms
- Soybeans
- Yogurt

*Tryptophan*

- Almonds
- Buckwheat flour
- Navy beans
- Soybean nuts
- Watermelon seeds
- Black beans
- Cottage cheese
- Seaweed
- Tofu
- Whole-wheat flower

*Dietary fiber*

- Black beans
- Chickpeas
- Figs
- Pinto beans
- Rye flour
- Bran cereals
- Corn bran
- Pears
- Refried beans
- Whole-wheat flour

*Omega-3 fatty acid*

- Canola oil
- Salmon
- Soybean oil
- Tofu
- Walnuts
- Flaxseed
- Soy milk
- Soybeans
- Walnut oil
- Wheat germ

Now that we have identified some physical strategies for managing head pain, let's look closely at a vital area to our well-being: our emotional and spiritual condition. We are made up of body, mind, *and* spirit, and in treating headache symptoms we cannot divorce one area from the other three. We will take a closer look at the psychological and spiritual strategies to relieve headache pain.

CHAPTER 12

# Psychological and Spiritual Strategies for Headache Relief

*There is no medicine like hope, no incentive so great, and no tonic so powerful as expectation of something better tomorrow.*[1]

—Orison Marden

In seeking to experience optimal health, it is important to remember that you cannot separate the mind from the body. They are one, and they have a strong influence on each other. If you are experiencing physical difficulties (like headaches), it will begin to influence your thinking and emotions. If you are having emotional difficulties or your thinking is negative, it will eventually affect your physical health.

Any type of pain—whether it is physical or emotional—is sending a message. It is important that we attempt to determine the source of that message or the purpose of the message. Pain is a wake-up call to say that something is wrong. The pain message might be saying, "You are under too much stress." It could be saying, "You are not eating right." It might be shouting, "You are not working out like you should. You need to exercise." The headache message might be alerting you to damaged or broken relationships.

Dr. Oliver Sacks has made an interesting observation about migraine headaches. Dr. Sacks is professor of neurology at the Albert Einstein College of Medicine in New York. He is also the author of a very comprehensive book on headaches simply titled *Migraine.* Dr. Sacks states:

> Some patients I could help with drugs, and some with the magic of attention and interest. The most severely afflicted patients defeated my therapeutic endeavors until I started to inquire minutely and persistently into their emotional lives. It now became apparent to me that many migraine attacks were drenched in emotional significance, and could not be usefully considered, let alone treated, unless their emotional antecedents and effects were exposed in detail.[2]

Dr. Sacks is suggesting that the elimination of headaches involves more than simply giving someone a pill. The pill only deals with the results or the symptoms. It does not address the source, or more likely, a combination of sources. In any type of healing process, one must remember to treat not only the problem but also the person.

The thinking process directly affects the physical body. If we have a positive attitude and outlook, we will feel good emotionally. How we feel affects our work and our health.

I am reminded of the story of two men digging a trench with shovels. One man was digging slowly and was uttering negative words about the work. The other man was digging with speed and great enthusiasm. A passerby asked, "What are you doing?"

The first man said, "Can't you see? We are digging a trench on a hot day! It's a lot of hard work, and I wish I was home relaxing and drinking a lemonade!"

The other man looked up, smiled, and said, "I'm helping to dig a trench for the foundation of a beautiful cathedral. I can't wait to see what it looks like!"

Throughout this book I have attempted to suggest that headaches may involve a complex interaction between what we eat, our working conditions, the air we breathe, our physical exercise, the stress we are under, and our attitude. For this reason, we may have to approach relieving headaches by a number of methods.

If we were to take your headache temperature potential, how would you rate? Would you register high in the optimal health area, or would you register low in some of the symptom (causal) areas? Using the chart below, place a check mark at the level you think you are at this point in time.

**OPTIMAL HEALTH CHART**

| | PERFECT | EXCELLENT | ADEQUATE | NEED TO IMPROVE | HOLDS ME BACK | POOR | CRITICAL |
|---|---|---|---|---|---|---|---|
| Physical | | | | | | | |
| Mental | | | | | | | |
| Emotional | | | | | | | |
| Social | | | | | | | |
| Spiritual | | | | | | | |
| Vocational | | | | | | | |
| Financial | | | | | | | |
| Friendships | | | | | | | |
| Gratitude | | | | | | | |
| Service | | | | | | | |
| Optimism | | | | | | | |
| Lifestyle | | | | | | | |
| Sense of humor | | | | | | | |

Are you happy where you are on this chart? Are there areas that need improvement? Do you think that certain categories contribute more to your headaches in any way? Let's take a closer look at some strategies that you can do to relieve headaches.

## ANGER REDUCTION

Nothing can destroy a relationship quicker than anger. It is a very powerful emotion that needs to be under control. Anger can affect the body by tightening the muscles of the head, neck, back, and stomach. Anger can bring about heart attacks. Anger can make almost any disease that affects the body worse. Anger can be the trigger or source for a terrific headache.

Aristotle said, "It is easy to fly into a passion—anybody can do that—but to be angry with the right person to the right extent and at the right time and with the right object and in the right way—that is not easy, and it is not everyone who can do it."[3]

To best control anger, it is important to understand it. Anger is a motivation. If harnessed, it can stand against injustice, crime, and corruption. If it is not harnessed, it will run like a wild bull in a china closet. It can destroy everything with which it comes into contact.

| ANGER CAN FIND ITS ROOTS IN... | | |
|---|---|---|
| Alcohol | Being angry at God | Body chemistry |
| Boredom | Criticism | Culture |
| Drugs | Ego | Embarrassment |
| Envy | Expectations | Fear of failure |
| Frustration | General stress | Helplessness |
| Humiliation | Injustice | Insecurity |
| Interpretations | Jealousy | Lack of privacy |
| Loss of a job | Loss of a loved one | Loss of health |
| Loss of love | Loss of respect | Modeling from family |
| Moods | Need for space | Past experiences |

| ANGER CAN FIND ITS ROOTS IN... | | |
|---|---|---|
| Perceptions | Physical disabilities | Physical injury |
| Protection of family | Rejection | Religious disappointment |
| Revenge | Selfishness | Sleep loss |
| Social pressure | Unfulfilled desires | Uselessness |
| Values | Weather conditions | |

To help you control your angry thoughts and feelings it is important to:

1. *Learn to discipline your mind.* Don't just say the first thing that comes to your thinking.

   **A gentle answer turns away wrath, *but a harsh word stirs up anger.***

   **—Proverbs 15:1, NIV, emphasis added**

2. *Don't put off expressing how you feel for long periods of time.* Garbage has a tendency to build up.

   **"In your anger do not sin:" Do not let the sun go down while you are still angry.**

   **—Ephesians 4:26, NIV**

3. *Nothing is solved by silence.* Make it a habit not to withdraw into silence.

4. *Be open to criticism.* This is difficult because we want to justify our actions and fight back when any type of attack comes.

   **Get rid of all bitterness, rage and anger, brawling and slander, along with every form of malice.**

   **—Ephesians 4:31, NIV**

5. *Share one issue at a time.* Don't back up the garbage truck and drop the entire load.

6. *Don't use the past to manipulate other people.* Beating people over the head with their past errors does not help the present or plan for the future.

   **An angry man stirs up dissension, and a hot-tempered one commits many sins.**

   **—PROVERBS 29:22, NIV**

7. *Learn to express your expectations for others verbally.* They don't have a crystal ball that tells them what you are thinking or what expectations you have for them.

   **My dear brothers, take note of this: Everyone should be quick to listen, slow to speak and slow to become angry, for man's anger does not bring about the righteous life that God desires.**

   **—JAMES 1:19–20, NIV**

8. *State your hurt or complaint as objectively as possible.* Use "I" words rather than "you" words. "You" words are aggressive and attacking. They only escalate the anger.

   **Starting a quarrel is like breaching a dam; so drop the matter before a dispute breaks out.**

   **—PROVERBS 17:14, NIV**

9. *Share your complaint in private, not in public.* Everyone, even you, wants to save face.

   **If your brother sins against you, go and show him his fault, just between the two of you.**

   **—MATTHEW 18:15, NIV**

10. *Don't throw the baby out with the bathwater.* Let the other party know that you are not dissatisfied with the entire relationship.

11. *Avoid a win-lose situation.* Rather than trying to conquer the other person, try to conquer the problem.

    **A patient man has great understanding, but a quick-tempered man displays folly.**

    **—PROVERBS 14:29, NIV**

12. *Don't make threats to terminate or leave the relationship.* They might just take you up on your offer. You may regret your big mouth.

13. *Don't always be joking.* Anger is not a laughing matter. Many jokes have deep anger hidden in them. "My wife, when she sits around the house, she sits *around* the house."

14. *Don't accuse or attack the other person.* Phrases like *you always, you never,* and *every time you* cause the angry emotions to rise.

    **A hot-tempered man stirs up dissension, but a patient man calms a quarrel.**

    **—PROVERBS 15:18, NIV**

15. *Look for a solution.* Seek reconciliation in all relationships if possible.

    **A man's wisdom gives him patience; it is his glory to overlook an offense.**

    **—PROVERBS 19:11, NIV**

16. *Allow for reaction time.* Some people cannot respond or come up with responses immediately. They need time to think it over. Give them a little space. Wouldn't you appreciate it if the shoe were on the other foot?

It is important to reduce angry emotions. Anger left unchecked only increases hurt feelings, tension, and many headaches. For a detailed presentation of anger reduction, may I suggest my book titled *Anger Is a Choice.*

## CONFLICT RESOLUTION

Conflict is a normal part of life. It occurs within the home, at school, in the workplace, around the community, all over the nation, and throughout the world.

When conflict is not dealt with, it begins to grow and becomes a monster that overpowers us.

When there is conflict between parents and children, brothers and sisters, or with relatives, the tension begins to mount. Damaged relationships on the job, in the church, and in the community can escalate to involve many people rather than just two adversaries.

Much time is spent in thinking about the conflict. Emotions can run high. Revenge can rear its ugly head. Harsh words can be spoken, and physical action has been known to break out.

To help reduce the conflict in relationships and the triggers that can cause headaches, it is good to get more information before you respond. Often we have misunderstood what someone has said or something that they have done. It is wise to get more facts before you end up "putting your foot in your mouth." The key to getting more facts is to ask strategic questions. Wise King Solomon said, "He who answers before listening—that is his folly and his shame" (Prov. 18:13, NIV).

Go to the memory file stored in your brain. Ask yourself, *Is this conflict similar to any other conflicts that I have had in the past? Does the person I'm having conflict with remind me of anyone out of my past? Am I bringing past events and emotions into a situation that is similar but entirely in a class by itself?*

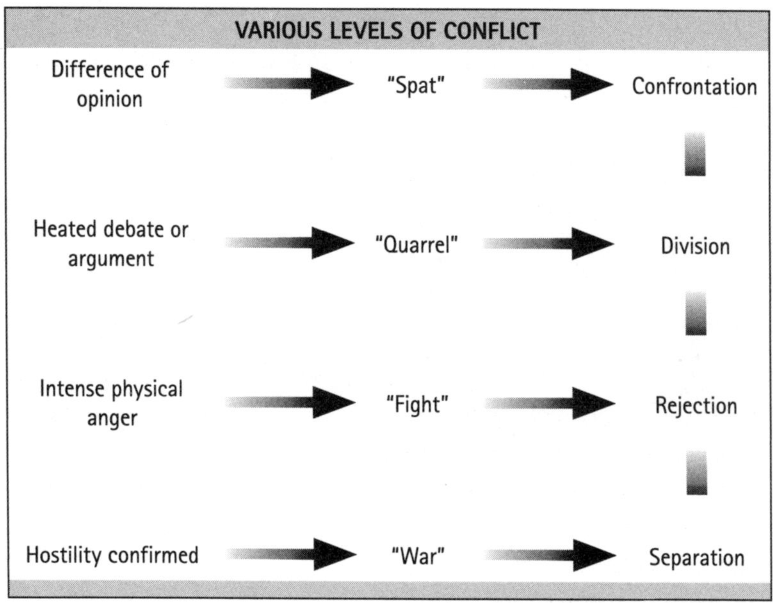


It is easy to have a displacement response and take out our frustrations on our spouse or children when we are really angry or upset with someone else. It is a way of venting at the wrong person. Cesare Pavese has suggested that, "Anger is never sudden. It is born out of a long, prior irritation that has ulcerated the spirit and built up an accumulation of force that results in an explosion. It follows that a fine outburst of rage is by no means a sign of a frank, direct nature."[5]

We can resolve conflict by using *power*—the power of aggression or withholding benefits. Or, we can resolve conflict by *demanding rights.* This will involve agreed-upon rules, contracts, or minutes. The best approach is to attempt to *reconcile interests.* This will take into consideration both parties' needs, values, and concerns. It has been said that for every interest involved, there usually exist several possible positions that could satisfy it. A key factor is respect for everyone's participation and suggestions.

Behind opposite positions lie many more compatible interests than conflicting ones. It is important to look for commonalties, interests, and solutions. The focus should be on future shared benefits for both parties.

Learn to face the conflict even if it is painful or difficult. To run from conflict will be a continual race.

For a detailed presentation of how to resolve conflict, may I suggest my book titled *How to Deal With Annoying People.*

## COUNSELING FOR INDIVIDUALS

If you have been plagued by past hurts, fears, anger, depression, compulsions, guilt, low self-image, and other emotional struggles—counseling may be beneficial for you. Sometimes it is helpful to have someone to navigate you through the complexities of life.

However, don't enter into counseling thinking that all of your problems will just disappear. Life is simply not that way. There is a combination of hurts and sorrows—and joys and laughter in life. As much as you would like to, you can't avoid suffering. At some point it will come. So what else is new?

Counseling helps one adjust to the realities of life. It helps us to learn to accept what we *can* change and make peace with what we *cannot* change. Human suffering has created some of the strongest souls. We don't remember people for the easy life they have led. We remember them for overcoming great obstacles. Abraham Lincoln did not have an easy life. Mahatma Gandhi faced great difficulties. Mother Teresa suffered many trials. We remember them for their positive character in the midst of daily struggle.

Emotional hurts, worries, and concerns can be the source for many headaches. We are not perfect. We fail often to reach our own goals and expectations. Guilt for past misdeeds can haunt us.

We can come from dysfunctional families that model poorly how to get along with others. Friends can disappoint us, health may fail, and true love may elude us. Join the human race.

When you are struggling with the pressures of life, it is often helpful to get outside help and advice. It is good to get different points of view when we face important decisions. Good advice will save us from reinventing the wheel and spending needless energy going in the wrong direction. Wise counsel will help to eliminate good ideas from bad ideas. It will help to crystallize our thinking and perspective.

When you seek a counselor, look for someone who has experience and is mature in his thinking. Ask yourself questions such as, *Can I trust him? Is he someone I would like to know? Do I respect him? Does he have a good reputation? Do I feel comfortable with him?*

Being comfortable with your counselor does not mean that he will only tell you things you want to hear. Often, the best counselor is one who will challenge your thinking and will be honest with you.

Sidney Harris said, "The most unrewarding task in the world is trying to tell people the truth about themselves before they are ready to hear it; and even Aesop, who cast such truth in fable form, was eventually thrown off a cliff because his morals struck too close to home."[6]

A good counselor will earn his or her money. It is not an easy task to deal all day with the emotional hurts of others. The counselor understands that change is not usually an overnight event. It is a process, and that process is sometimes painful. One counselor I know calls this process "Forming, Storming, Norming, and Performing."

- Forming: Explaining the details of the problem
- Storming: Going through the pain of growth
- Norming: Getting one's life back to normal

- Performing: Living a healthy life of doing what we should be doing

For a detailed presentation of the benefits of personal counseling, may I suggest my book titled *Getting Off the Emotional Roller Coaster.*

### FAMILY COUNSELING

Family counseling is a little different from personal counseling. The family counselor realizes that all families have unspoken systems of operation. These systems can be healthy or unhealthy.

For example, in some families everyone yells. That is what is familiar to them, that is what is comfortable for them, and that is the habit pattern they have established. When conflict comes to their family, they have a tendency to attack each other. On the other hand, some families are quiet. Everyone holds in their thoughts and feelings. They have a tendency to withdraw from each other during any conflict. Then there are those families that have mixed reactions of attack and withdraw during conflict.

Family counselors are also alert to the triangling that goes on in families. Triangling involves two of the members being on the inside and one member on the outside of family issues. This causes a polarization and escalation of conflict.

As conflict rises, so does tension. Headaches can be experienced by more than one person in the family.

Some headache studies indicate that people who have migraine headaches come from families that have migraines. This information is used to suggest that migraine headaches are hereditary. Family counselors will question that theory and suggest that headaches are not hereditary but are caused by the negative and hostile environment that everyone lives in. The latter theory is easier to prove than the former theory. It simply makes common sense that headaches arise when there is much emotional turmoil in the home, especially when the home is supposed to be a place of safety and retreat from a hostile world.

When families come in for counseling, they come with a sense of failure. They realize that there is a crisis in their home. The Chinese word for *crisis* is made up of two symbols. One symbol represents danger, and the other symbol represents opportunity. A family crisis is a dangerous opportunity. Family counselors will attempt to help the family identify the opportunity in the crisis.

Family counselors are also aware that families may have an escalation of conflict for a short period of time as a result of counseling. Long-denied family agony may come to the surface. This is because their traditional family system is being shaken up and challenged. The whole family will struggle for a period as they learn a new system of communication with each other. No one likes change. They will all have a tendency to resist the new and unfamiliar. The only one who likes change is a newborn baby.

The family counselor is also alert to determine if conflict is being generated by the situation in the home, intrapersonal problems within an individual member, or interpersonal problems between certain family members.

## FORGIVENESS

Harboring bitterness, resentment, and unforgiveness can emotionally destroy a person. Over time, these emotions can be the cause for numerous headaches. Unforgiveness does not solve anything. It only stifles and brings misery to the person who will not forgive.

Have you ever wondered why forgiveness is so difficult? It is because the person who has been injured does the forgiving—and lets the injurer go free. The person injured gets no repayment and no revenge, and all he ends up with is resentment. This is a dirty deal.

You may say, "But I don't *feel* like forgiving them." Well, I have news for you. Forgiveness is not a feeling first. How do I know that? Because it will be a cold day in the hot place before I *feel* like forgiving you, you dirty dog. You've hurt me.

True forgiveness involves three major factors:

1. *I will not use it against them in the future.* I won't beat them over the head with the past.
2. *I will not talk to others about them.* I know that misery loves company, but I will make a determined effort not to bad-mouth them to other people.
3. *I will not dwell on it myself.* This is the hardest part of forgiveness. I simply have to just let go of it. I need to bury the hatchet and not draw a map to the burial sight so I can dig it up later.

Is there someone in your life whom you haven't forgiven? Let me ask you a question. Has harboring all your resentment helped the situation? Do you feel any better for it?

I'm reminded of the man who goes to his doctor and says, "Doctor, every time I lift my arm it hurts."

The doctor responded, "So don't lift it."

> Stop being mean, bad-tempered, and angry. Quarreling, harsh words, and dislike of others should have no place in your lives. Instead, be kind to each other, tenderhearted, forgiving one another, just as God has forgiven you because you belong to Christ.
>
> —Ephesians 4:31–32, TLB

Since unforgiveness only destroys the one holding it, why not try giving it up? It isn't working, is it? It only brings on headaches. Why continue to do something that only brings pain to yourself?

## PERSONALITY STYLES

Through the years there has been discussion of whether or not there is a "migraine personality." Are there personality traits or social styles of behaving that seem to have more headaches than others?

People who tend to be perfectionists have a higher incidence of headaches. This may be because they never can quite live up to the perfectionist standard and are frustrated, which triggers headaches. It may be because they have a hard time saying no or have the inability to delegate responsibility. They don't want to lose control and have something done wrong.

There are four basic social styles. They are the Analyticals, the Drivers, the Amiables, and the Expressives. I personally believe that they all can have headaches, and if they do not personally have them, they can give them to others by the way they behave.

Analyticals and Drivers are basically task oriented. Accomplishing tasks is a high priority for them. When this does not occur, they can become frustrated and uptight. This tension of not being able to complete tasks can trigger headaches.

Amiables and Expressives, on the other hand, are basically relationship oriented. When they cannot be with people as they desire, they can become irritated because they are forced to do tasks. This tension can also lead to headaches.

Let's take a moment and look at each social style individually. As we look at how they behave and what motivates them, it becomes clear that they will respond to headaches slightly differently.

| GENERAL OVERVIEW OF THE FOUR SOCIAL STYLES | | | | |
|---|---|---|---|---|
| AREA | ANALYTICALS | DRIVERS | AMIABLES | EXPRESSIVES |
| Reaction | Slow | Swift | Unhurried | Rapid |
| Orientation | Thinking and fact | Action and goal | Relationship and peace | Involvement and intuition |
| Likes | Organization | To be in charge | Close relationships | Much interaction |
| Dislikes | Involvement | Inaction | Conflict | To be alone |
| Maximum effort | To organize | To control | To relate | To involve |
| Minimum concern | For relationships | For caution in relationships | For effecting change | For routine |
| Behavior directed toward achievement | Works carefully and alone—primary effort | Works quickly and alone—primary effort | Works slowly and with others—secondary effort | Works quickly and with team—secondary effort |
| Behavior directed toward acceptance | Impresses others with precision and knowledge—secondary | Impresses others with individual effort—secondary | Gets along as integral member of group—primary | Gets along as exciting member of group—primary |
| Actions | Cautious | Decisive | Slow | Impulsive |
| Skills | Good problem-solving skills | Good administrative skills | Good counseling skills | Good persuasive skills |
| Decision making | Avoids risks, based on facts | Takes risks, based on intuition | Avoids risks, based on opinion | Takes risks, based on hunches |
| Use of time | Slow, deliberate, disciplined | Swift, efficient, impatient | Slow, calm, undisciplined | Rapid, quick, undisciplined |

As we look more specifically at the weaknesses of the four social styles, it will become clear that they will respond to tension and pressure in their own unique way.

| ANALYTICAL | |
|---|---|
| **WHAT THEY VALUE** | **WHAT ANNOYS THEM** |
| • Security | • Inaccuracy |
| • Accuracy | • Incompetence |
| • Stability | • Change |
| • Rules and regulations | • Aggressiveness |
| • Quality | • Shouting |
| • Structure | • Evasiveness |
| • Efficiency | • Mediocrity |
| • Facts | • Inadequacy |
| • Competence | • Exaggeration |
| • Details | • Invasiveness |
| • Tradition | • Clutter |
| • Critical thinking | • Disorganization |
| • Organization | • Clamor |
| • Logic | • Hastiness |

### THE ANALYTICAL'S WEAKNESSES

*Snapshot of the Analytical*

- Remembers the negative
- Moody and depressed
- Enjoys being hurt
- False humility
- Off in another world
- Low self-image
- Selective hearing
- Self-centered
- Too introspective
- Guilt feelings
- Persecution complex
- Tends to be a hypochondriac

*The Analytical at work*

- Not people oriented
- Depressed over imperfections
- Chooses difficult work
- Hesitant to start projects
- Spends too much time planning
- Prefers analysis to actual work
- Hard to please
- Self-deprecating
- Standards often too high
- Deep need for approval

*The Analytical as a parent*

- Puts goals beyond reach
- May discourage children
- May be too meticulous
- Becomes a martyr
- Sulks over disagreements
- Puts guilt on children

*The Analytical as a friend*

- Lives through others
- Withdrawn and remote
- Socially insecure
- Critical of others
- Holds back affection
- Dislikes those in opposition
- Suspicious of people
- Antagonistic and vengeful
- Unforgiving
- Full of contradictions
- Skeptical of compliments

| DRIVERS | |
|---|---|
| **WHAT THEY VALUE** | **WHAT ANNOYS THEM** |
| • Achievement | • Indecisiveness |
| • Challenge | • Boredom |
| • Success | • Small talk |
| • Power | • Details |
| • Speed | • Hypersensitivity |
| • Control | • Over-emotional |
| • Responsibility | • Dependency |
| • Goals | • Excuses |
| • Debates | • Irresponsibility |
| • Competition | • Lethargy |
| • Leadership | • Laziness |
| • Independence | • Procrastination |
| • Decisiveness | • Taking orders |
| • Productivity | • Over-analyzing |

## THE DRIVER'S WEAKNESSES

*Snapshot of the Driver*

- Bossy
- Impatient
- Quick-tempered
- Can't relax
- Too impetuous
- Enjoys controversy and arguments
- Won't give up when losing
- Comes on too strong
- Inflexible
- Not complimentary
- Dislikes tears and emotions
- Is unsympathetic

*The Driver at work*

- Little tolerance for mistakes
- Demands loyalty in ranks

- Doesn't analyze details
- Bored by trivia
- May make rash decisions
- May be rude or tactless
- Manipulates people
- Demanding of others
- End justifies means
- Work may become god

*The Driver as a parent*

- Tends to overdominate
- Too busy for family
- Gives answers too quickly
- Impatient with poor performance
- Won't let children relax
- May send them into depression

*The Driver as a friend*

- Tends to use people
- Dominates others
- Decides for others
- Knows everything
- Can do everything better
- Is too independent
- Possessive of friends and mate
- Can't say "I'm sorry"

| AMIABLES | |
|---|---|
| **WHAT THEY VALUE** | **WHAT ANNOYS THEM** |
| • Contribution | • Conflict |
| • Comfort | • Impatience |
| • Compassion | • Disrespect |
| • Cooperation | • Discourteousness |
| • Friendliness | • Insensitivity |
| • Peacefulness | • Harshness |
| • Loyalty | • Rushing |
| • Approval | • Pressure |
| • Cohesiveness | • Tension |
| • Trust | • Controversy |
| • Kindness | • Disharmony |
| • Relationships | • Yelling |
| • Benevolence | • Pushiness |
| • Coaching | • Rudeness |

## THE AMIABLE'S WEAKNESSES

*Snapshot of the Amiable*

- Unenthusiastic
- Fearful and worried
- Indecisive
- Avoids responsibility
- Quiet will of iron
- Selfish
- Too shy and reticent
- Too compromising
- Self-righteous

*The Amiable at work*

- Not goal-oriented
- Lacks self-motivation
- Hard to get moving
- Resents being pushed
- Lazy and careless

- Discourages others
- Would rather watch

*The Amiable as a parent*

- Lax on discipline
- Doesn't organize the home
- Takes life too easily
- Will ignore family conflict

*The Amiable as a friend*

- Dampens enthusiasm
- Stays uninvolved
- Is not exciting
- Indifferent to plans
- Judges others
- Sarcastic and teasing
- Resists change

| EXPRESSIVES | |
|---|---|
| **WHAT THEY VALUE** | **WHAT ANNOYS THEM** |
| • Freedom | • Rules |
| • Excitement | • Structure |
| • Adventure | • Schedules |
| • Flexibility | • Routine |
| • Spontaneity | • Tedium |
| • Vision | • Stagnation |
| • Enthusiasm | • Slowness |
| • Change | • Boredom |
| • Unpredictability | • Ritual |
| • Uniqueness | • Unoriginal |
| • Creativity | • Uncreative |
| • Innovation | • Details |
| • Versatility | • Formality |

## THE EXPRESSIVE'S WEAKNESSES

*Snapshot of the Expressive*

- Compulsive talker
- Exaggerates and elaborates
- Dwells in trivia
- Can't remember names
- Scares others off
- Too happy for some people
- Restless energy
- Egotistical
- Blusters and complains
- Naïve and gullible
- Loud voice and laugh
- Controlled by circumstances
- Angers easily
- Seems phony to some people
- Never grows up

*The Expressive at work*

- Would rather talk
- Forgets obligations
- Doesn't follow through
- Confidence fades fast
- Undisciplined
- Priorities out of order
- Decides by feelings
- Easily distracted
- Wastes time talking

*The Expressive as a parent*

- Keeps home in a frenzy
- Forgets children's appointments
- Disorganized
- Doesn't listen to the whole story

*The Expressive as a friend*

- Hates to be alone
- Needs to be center stage
- Wants to be popular
- Looks for credit
- Dominates conversations
- Interrupts and doesn't listen
- Answers for others
- Fickle and forgetful
- Makes excuses
- Repeats stories

Your personality style will determine to some degree the frequency and intensity of your headaches. Your attitude and how you view problems and difficulties are a strategic issue. How do you view your problems? Do you look at them with a positive or negative attitude? Do you see the glass half full or half empty? Do you see a rose with every thorn or a thorn with every rose? Do you see an opportunity in every difficulty or a difficulty in every opportunity? Do you see endless hope or a hopeless ending? Do you see obstacles, or do you see challenges?

> And now, brothers, as I close this letter, let me say this one more thing: Fix your thoughts on what is true and good and right. Think about things that are pure and lovely, and dwell on the fine, good things in others. Think about all you can praise God for and be glad about. Keep putting into practice all you learned from me and saw me doing, and the God of peace will be with you.
>
> —Philippians 4:8–9, TLB

## RELAXATION AND VISUALIZATION

Many headaches are related to muscle tension in various portions of the body. Muscle tension can be eased through the use of relaxation and visualization.

The following exercises can be done twice a day for a ten- to twenty-minute period of time. It is ideal to have a quiet room where you can turn down the lights and play soft music. However, the same exercises can be done without the dim lights and soft music.

1. Lie on the floor on your back.
2. Place a pillow under your neck, filling the gap that is normally created when lying down.
3. Place a pillow under your legs on the backside of the knees. Have your hands comfortably lying at your sides.
4. Close your eyes and begin to slowly breathe in and out. Breathe in to the count of six. Hold your breath for the count of six. Let out your breath to the count of six. With each breath in, energy enters the body. With each breath out, tension leaves the body. Concentrate on breathing in and out for about twenty exhales.
5. Next, make a fist and tightly squeeze each hand. Hold the fist for a count of six. Then spread out your fingers as far as you can to the count of six. Do that three times, and then relax your hands entirely.
6. Next, contract your arm muscles to the count of six, and relax them similar to the hands. Tighten your arms three times, and then relax.
7. Next, contract both of your legs in the same way you tightened your arms—hold for a count of six and then relax. Do it three times.

8. Next, contract your stomach muscles in similar fashion.
9. Next, contract your chest muscles in similar fashion.
10. Next, contract your shoulder muscles in similar fashion.
11. Next, contract your neck muscles in similar fashion.
12. Finally, contract your face and head muscles in similar fashion.
13. When you are finished contacting and relaxing muscles, let your entire body relax. Concentrate on breathing in and out normally—not keeping a six count. Energy comes in on the inhale, and tension goes out on the exhale.
14. Now, begin to imagine your favorite spot. It could be at the beach. It might be in the mountains. You may prefer an island getaway or floating in a hot-air balloon. Visualize the spot in your mind. You may want to feel the warmth of the sun on your body or the coolness of water. It is up to you. Whichever spot you select, begin to visualize what you see in detail. What sounds would you like to hear? What smells would you like to smell? What would you like to feel? Imagine these things, and continue to relax deeper with each breath.
15. It is good to determine how much time you have to spend in relaxation before you begin the exercise. If it is fifteen minutes, ask your body to remind you when it is time to get up. Our bodies

have an amazing ability to keep very accurate time. When it comes time to end your relaxation and visualization period, take ten last relaxing breaths and then get up. You will be amazed at how refreshed you will feel.

### SPIRITUAL COUNSELING AND YOUR SOUL

When it comes to spiritual counseling, there seems to be three categories of people.

1. **The "Whatevers."** These are those who couldn't care less about spiritual matters. They do not have any background in religious faith and do not feel a need to develop one. Or, if they do have some previous knowledge, they have chosen to reject it for various reasons.
2. **The "Ah-ahs!"** These are those who may or may not have some spiritual background but are interested in the topic. They are seekers who are open to consider this avenue of life and would like further information.
3. **The Thinkers.** These are those who are deeply concerned about spiritual matters. Their emotional and mental health are tied closely to their faith and how it affects their daily life. They strive, in various degrees, to attempt to grow in their faith and knowledge.

Those who are interested or are deeply concerned about spiritual matters identify with the words of Jesus when He says, "For what profit is it to a man if he gains the whole world, and loses his own soul? Or what will a man give in exchange for his soul?" (Matt. 16:26).

Jesus is simply saying that there is more to life than just material goods. He suggests that it is dangerous not to consider the deeper purposes of life. Have you ever wondered what life is all about? Have you ever questioned why there is pain and suffering...and why there are headaches? Have you ever wondered if God has a plan for your life?

You see, life is not always an easy road. Sometimes we encounter the potholes of difficulties, the pain of bumps, the detours of depression, and the roughness of headaches. During these times of discomfort, it is easy to become weary of it all. Are you tired and weary of the pressures in your life and the various troubles you face? Then join the club. Many people feel the same way.

Spiritual counseling suggests that God does care about you and the problems you face. God wants to come to your aid and help you through the tough times that cause headaches.

Jesus said, "Come to Me, all you who labor and are heavy laden, and I will give you rest. Take My yoke upon you and learn from Me, for I am gentle and lowly in heart, and you will find rest for your souls. For My yoke is easy and My burden is light" (Matt. 11:28–30).

How does one come to Jesus? How does a person find rest for his soul? How can I experience peace (less headaches) in the midst of turmoil? Jesus said, "Peace I leave with you, My peace I give to you; not as the world gives do I give to you. Let not your heart be troubled, neither let it be afraid" (John 14:27).

To experience peace with God, and the peace of God, starts with understanding who Jesus is. While on earth, He was God in a human body. He came to tell us how to have a relationship with Him that would last for eternity.

When our Pointman Leadership Institute Team held a leadership seminar in Mongolia, a professor of literature who was a parliament member said to me, "I don't understand your God. He has three faces—Father, Son, and Holy Spirit. How can that be?" The following conversation then ensued:

"You are a professor of literature, are you not?"

"Yes, I am."

"Is the name Shakespeare familiar to you?"

"Of course."

"Are you acquainted with the character Macbeth?"

"Yes, I am."

"May I ask you a question? Could the character Macbeth ever meet the author, Shakespeare?"

He thought for a moment and replied, "No, he could not."

"Ahhh, but he could. All the author would have to do is to write himself into the play and then introduce himself to Macbeth. That's what God (the Father) did when He wrote Himself into the play of life in the form of the Son (Jesus of Nazareth). He became the God/man."

God is a perfect and holy being. We as humans are not perfect because we have imperfections. Try as we may, we often fall short of doing the right thing, saying the right thing, or thinking the right thing. Do you know anyone who is perfect?

This imperfection, or sin, is what separates us from a holy God. Now God has a problem, because He loves us. He chooses to deal with our sinfulness—our imperfections. His Son was sent to die in our place, pay our penalty, and buy us back from the slave market of sinfulness and wickedness.

Jesus bore our sins on the cross for us. He died in our place. He was buried for our cruelty and rose from the grave to establish a new life and relationship with God for us. All we have to do is to have faith in Him.

The apostle Paul states it this way: "That if you confess with your mouth the Lord Jesus and believe in your heart that God has raised Him from the dead, you will be saved. For with the heart one believes unto righteousness, and with the mouth confession is made unto salvation.... For whoever calls on the name of the Lord shall be saved" (Rom. 10:9–10, 13).

Have you prayed before to receive Christ? If not, you can do it right now. Just put down this book and pray a simple prayer of faith asking Jesus to come into your life. Thank Him for dying in your place. Thank Him for providing a new relationship with God. Ask God to bring people into your life who will help you to grow and learn more about Him. Thank Him for saving you.

When you invite Jesus to come into your life, God sends His Holy Spirit to dwell within. He will be there to teach you about God. He will support you in tough times. He will help you to endure pain and suffering (even headaches), and He will teach and lead you to learn how to lessen the frequency and severity of headaches.

To encourage you in the decision you just made, I would suggest that you look up the following verses in the Bible: John 6:37; Romans 10:9–13; Colossians 1:14, 27; Hebrews 13:5; 1 John 5:11–13; and Revelation 3:20.

What did you learn from these verses?

..............................................................................................................

..............................................................................................................

..............................................................................................................

..............................................................................................................

Read the Bible every day. Following is a very simple daily Bible study plan.

1. Select one of the books within the Bible that you would like to read. A good book to start with would be the Gospel of John, the fourth book in the New Testament.

2. Read one chapter a day until you are finished with that book.

3. As you read each chapter make some notes. Try and identify the following: (a) the key verse of the chapter (central thought); (b) God's com-

mands (a command is something to do); (c) God's promises (a promise is something to be believed); (d) a short summary of the chapter; and (e) personal applications you received from reading that particular chapter that you can apply to your daily life.

4.Look up 1 Peter 2:2 and Psalm 119:9, 11.

Talk to God daily (prayer) and keep your relationship with Him growing. Read 1 John 1:9; Psalm 66:18; and Philippians 4:6–7.

Fellowship with other believers. Get involved in a local church where the truth about Jesus is taught. (See Hebrews 10:25.)

Begin to tell others about Jesus. Learn to serve God wherever you can. Help others grow in their faith. Look up Matthew 28:19–20; Mark 5:19; Acts 1:8; Ephesians 4:29; and 1 Corinthians 10:31. What did you learn from reading these Bible verses?

.................................................................................................

.................................................................................................

.................................................................................................

.................................................................................................

To help you to grow spiritually, I have included a Scripture index for various life topics. This index can be found at the back of the book. May your soul be refreshed as you study the Word of God.

CHAPTER 13

# Miscellaneous Strategies for Headache Relief

*If we could give every individual the right amount of nourishment and exercise, not too little and not too much, we would have found the safest way to health.*[1]

—HIPPOCRATES

As we near the end of this book, I have included various headache strategies that may be helpful for you. See if you can find any that may be of assistance in helping to reduce the headaches in your life.

## HIGH ALTITUDE

In chapter five, there was the suggestion that some people get headaches as they move from sea level to higher altitudes. At sea level the body adjusts to the weight of the air (pressure) on the body. As one rises in altitude, the air becomes lighter, and depending how high one goes, there is less oxygen. The decrease of oxygen (less pressure) causes the blood vessels of the brain to expand to compensate for the shortage of oxygen. This expansion irritates the nerves and brings on a headache.

When you travel in an airplane, the airlines pressurize the cabins where the passengers sit to make up for the lack of oxygen. If they did not do that, you would most likely pass out.

When we went to La Paz, Bolivia, we were told that the altitude might be difficult for us. The city is located at an altitude of 12,795 feet above sea level. It was suggested that we take aspirin for about a week before we arrived to help thin our blood a little. This would assist us in our adjustment to the higher altitude.

If you are traveling to higher altitudes, aspirin may help you diminish the onset of a headache. When you reach the higher altitude, it is recommended that you do not do strenuous activity for a couple of days. This will allow your body to readjust to the change in air pressure.

### HORMONES

Many women experience headaches in relationship to their hormones. As they reach the peak of their menstrual cycle, fluctuations in estrogen occur. These changes in their hormones can bring about cramps, vomiting, and headaches. If these symptoms are severe, it is best to go to your physician and seek help.

With regard to oral contraceptives, it is a mixed bag. Some women experience headaches because of taking the pills. On the other hand, some women who have had headaches in the past find that their headaches diminish when they are on the pill.

It has been estimated that 60 percent of headaches in women can be linked to their menstrual cycle and the decrease of estrogen.[2]

Many women who battle headaches find that they disappear during the first trimester of their pregnancy, but they may return postpartum.

If you are experiencing headaches that you believe are linked to your hormone level, you may want to consult with your physician about alternative methods to adjust the estrogen level in your body.

### LIGHT—SUN

Bright light from the sun or from man-made sources can trigger headaches. We all have experienced the squinting of our eyes as we walk out of a darkened building into bright and glaring daylight. The muscles around our eyes tighten, and tension is the result. The light is almost painful because of its brightness.

Those who work in machine shops where welding is done may develop headaches. Flickering fluorescent lights, television and computer screens, and flash cameras can bring about headaches. The reflection of light off of shiny surfaces or bright headlights is also very irritating to the eyes and can trigger headaches.

The use of sunglasses can help to diminish glare and reduce light-producing headaches. If you have fluorescent lights that flicker, it is important to change the electrical ballast or replace the fluorescent lights with the more stable incandescent light bulbs.

## NOISE

We live in a society where it is difficult to escape from noise. The honking of horns, screech of sirens, and blare of loud music is everywhere. Many people have to work in factories that are filled with noisy machinery, power tools, and pneumatic drills.

Plane, train, and automobile noises are common. Some people even put large boom-box speakers in their cars and trucks. Even with *your* car windows rolled up you can hear the throbbing bass of the music in other vehicles. In fact, you can even physically feel the sound waves from powerful subwoofers.

You cannot eliminate or control many of the sounds around you. You can, however, learn to carry earplugs with you when you travel or when you go to the place where you work.

## OXYGEN

Air quality is very beneficial for optimal health. It has been estimated that over one million hospital admissions a year are related to poor air quality. Various forms of smog and air pollution are major problems in many communities throughout the United States and other countries of the world. The poor air quality can be a trigger for headaches. Air quality is influenced by many sources. They include:

| | | |
|---|---|---|
| Aluminum dust | Animal dander | Asbestos |
| Automobile exhaust | Bacteria | Chromium (cement) |
| Coal fumes | Cobalt (cement) | Deodorizers |
| Dust | Dyes | Factory smoke |
| Fluorocarbons | Fog | Formalin |
| Fumes | Glues | Grain dusts |
| Grasses | Human hair | Insecticides |
| Mists | Molds | Motor oil |
| Oil smokes | Organophosphates | Paints |
| Particles (frayed) | Perfumes | Plant spores |
| Platinum salts / acids | Pollen | Polyvinyl chloride |
| Radon | Solvents | Tobacco smoke |
| Viruses | Wood dust | Yeast cells |

If the outdoor air quality is poor, it is recommended that you exercise inside. Jogging on a smoggy day next to the street where exhaust from cars, trucks, and buses spew into the air is not a wise decision. It could be the equivalent of smoking cigarettes.

If you work around dust, fumes, or smoke, you might be wise to wear some form of protective breathing mask. The various fumes might not affect you immediately, but they have a building residual component to them.

To help insure positive air quality, it is important to clean air ducts and change air filters. When was the last time you changed your air filters? Many new filters can eliminate very small particles in the air. Cleaning your carpets helps to diminish dust, dander, and various particles that cause allergies and breathing problems. Or better yet, replace carpet with tile or hardwood floors. Sometimes the chemicals in the carpet only aggravate respiratory problems. You may find the addition of live green plants helps improve the air quality.

You might consider purchasing a negative-ion generator for your home or place of business. These generators clean the air and leave that fresh smell that follows a rainstorm. Ionizers can remove particles from the air as small as .001 micron in size. This would include viruses, molds, dust, pollen, and cigarette smoke. They cost only pennies a month to operate.

It is estimated that we breathe about 23,000 times a day. Much of this breathing is shallow rather than deep. Shallow breathing does not bring sufficient oxygen into the body. One of the first signs of not taking in enough oxygen is the onset of headaches. They are tied together. In fact, studies of individuals who experience cluster headaches have found that breathing in oxygen for about fifteen minutes eliminates their headaches in most cases.

To practice deep breathing, lie down on the floor or a bed. Draw your knees up and allow them to spread apart slightly. Begin to relax and breathe deeply. Slowly draw in your breath to the count of six. Hold your breath for the count of six. Then slowly let your breath out to the count of six.

To assist you in breathing deeply, place a book on your stomach. As you breathe in, do it with the abdominal muscles causing the book to rise. As you breathe out, the book will fall with the lowering of your stomach. If you want to practice breathing deeply while sitting up—place both of your hands on your stom-

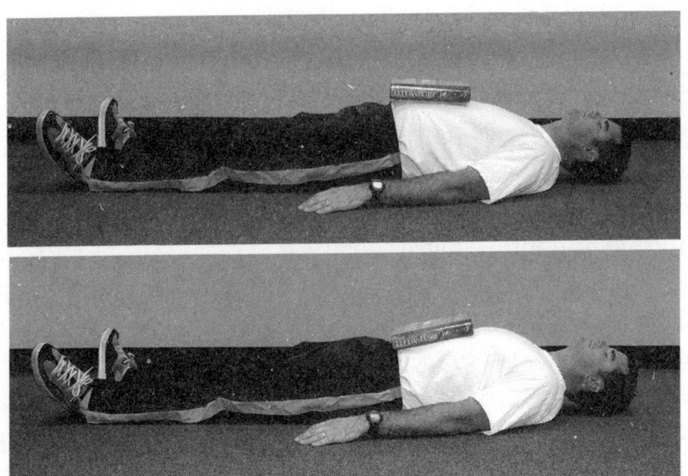

ach and slowly breathe in and out to the count of six as if you were lying on the floor. By having your hands on your stomach, you can feel if you are breathing deeply.

If you want to have a good exchange of air while you are walking, change your count a little. As you breathe in, count to four. Only this will not be a slow drawing in of air. It will be drawn in with four short separate inhales. You will not hold your breath. Immediately after drawing in the fourth breath, exhale to the count of four with four short separate exhales.

If you are running and want a good exchange of air, change your breathing count to two. Two quick separate inhales, followed by two quick separate exhales. The breathing in and out to the count of two will give you sufficient air while you are running and will help you to run longer distances. Counting to two—in and out—will help you to concentrate on your breathing rather than your running. You won't run very far if you are out of oxygen in your system.

### SINUSES

Many people suffer from sinus problems caused by allergies or illness.

This nasal inflammation is called allergic rhinitis. The blood vessels become swollen and inflamed. Congestion and pressure build. Stuffiness and postnasal drip begin. It is very uncomfortable and makes the individual feel below par. Often headaches of varying degrees emerge.

Sinus problems can be affected by perfumes, tobacco smoke, cleaning products, molds, mildews, pollen, dust, and a host of other impurities in the air. Sinuses can also be inflamed because of allergic reactions to feathers, cat dander, wheat, chocolate, hay, Bermuda grass, sugar, and milk products, just to name a few.

Ever since I was a small boy I had sinus problems. My nose was constantly running. I always had to carry a handkerchief with me wherever I went. The handkerchief was always damp from my blowing my nose.

One day I was talking to my chiropractor about my sinus problems. I told him about my constant drainage. He asked me two questions: "How much milk do you drink?" and "How much sugar do you eat?"

Well, I was drinking about a quart of milk with each meal and eating quite a few sweets. He suggested that I change what I was doing. I immediately went home and went "cold turkey" on the milk. I also cut back on the sweets, which was harder.

Within two weeks I saw dramatic improvement in my sinus drainage problem. After about two months, I ceased carrying a handkerchief with me. For the past twenty-six years, I have been virtually free of sinus drainage (other than an occasional cold).

Once in a while, I will take a small amount of low-fat milk with cereal. I still have to work on the sweets, but vast progress has been made.

Many times sinus problems are the result of taking too many nasal decongestants, antihistamines, steroid sprays, and sinus irrigations. They have a tendency to set up a rebound problem, similar as mentioned on pages 137–139.

How many decongestants and antihistamines are you taking? Maybe you would find relief by getting off of them, changing your diet, cleaning up your environment, and working on preventative measures. It's worth a try.

## SMOKING

I want to approach breaking the smoking habit because it might help eliminate your headaches if you smoke or if you are around smokers. It has been estimated that 90 percent of those who have cluster headaches are heavy smokers. Smoking increases the LDL (bad cholesterol) in your bloodstream. LDL encourages platelet clustering that can help to cause headaches.

Many heavy smokers with migraines report a decrease in headaches after they quit smoking. Oxygen is restored to the brain. Coughing from smoking diminishes, which helps to reduce the coughing trigger for headaches.

Those who have headaches and stop smoking may experience an increase of headache pain for a short time. This is a normal withdrawal reaction to the loss of nicotine in the bloodstream.

Dr. Ellen Grant published a study for the *Lancet* that involved thirty smokers. It studied their headache pattern before and after quitting smoking for thirty days.[3]

| THIRTY SMOKERS | MIGRAINES | HEADACHES | DAILY HEADACHES |
|---|---|---|---|
| Before (smoking) | 169 | 380 | 12 |
| After (not smoking) | 16 | 71 | 1 |

Let me drop in another argument for ceasing to smoke. It has nothing to do with the staining of teeth or the damaging of clothes. I won't address smoking from a moral point of view. I have a friend that says, “Smoking won't send you to hell; it just makes it smell like you have been there.”

There has been much discussion about the effects of cigarette smoking and lung cancer. Those arguments do not sway some cigarette smokers, who continue to smoke. The immediate gratification seems to outweigh the long-term results.

I can give you all the strategies known for overcoming headaches, but ultimately it is up to *you* to take action that will bring about change in your life.

# Conclusion

*All change represents loss of some kind... it is inconvenient, that's why we resist it so strongly.*[1]

*No man is free who is not a master of himself.*[2]

—EPICTETUS

Men of science and medicine, and even common sense, instruct us that headaches are the result of some cause. Headaches are not an illness. They are simply *a symptom* of something else going on. A true disease or illness like diabetes or a fever can create a platform for a headache to emerge, but the headache does not cause the disease. It is *a result* of the disease. Microorganisms do not enter my body carrying the "headache disease." There is no parasite or bacteria that carry tension-producing qualities. There are no viruses that carry the dreaded migraine headache.

Headaches come as a result of a number of factors like the environment, our physical health, foods we eat, exercise we get, medications we take, the stress we encounter, and even our attitude toward life. The combination of the various circumstances to which we are exposed, how we think and perceive things, and our reactions to them have a compounding effect. As these life stressors increase, a headache emerges. Headaches are the "straw that breaks the camel's back" or "the grain of sand that sinks the ship."

When headaches are experienced, sufferers have only one thought in mind: they want relief. They want to get rid of the pain immediately. This is usually accomplished by taking some form of pain medication. When the head pain is gone, headache sufferers then return to their normal activities. They are often too busy to question, "What brought about the headache in the first place?" Rarely does the person ask, "Is there a way to prevent headaches or at least reduce them?"

It has been the experience of many professionals in the field of medicine and psychology that people only change their behaviors when they *hurt enough*, are *scared enough*, or are *angry enough*. The overweight individual keeps on stuffing his or her body until the doctor says, "You're going to have a heart attack." Fear then motivates a change. The person who has back problems may not exercise and stretch muscles until he is physically tired of all the pain. The person in a dead-end job will not seek to better himself until he is upset enough with the circumstances to change. Anger will motivate him.

To drive home this point, let me share with you a passage from my book entitled *Getting Off the Emotional Roller Coaster.*

> I am reminded of a story that James MacDonald shares in his book, *I Really Want to Change.* It is the story of Raynald, who was a fourteenth-century duke in Belgium. Raynald eventually became the king of Belgium, but his brother Edward was very jealous.
>
> Edward convinced a group to follow him, and they overthrew Raynald's kingship. But Edward had compassion for Raynald and did not put him to death. Instead, he designed a special dungeon for him. It was a large circular room with one regular-sized doorway. It was outfitted with a bed, a table, and a chair. He

> included all the essentials that Raynald would need to be fairly comfortable.
>
> When the dungeon was completely built around Raynald, Edward paid him a visit. Edward pointed to the regular-sized doorway and called Raynald's attention to the fact that there was no door in the opening. A door was not necessary to keep Raynald in the dungeon because he was grossly overweight and too fat to squeeze through the opening. Edward then said to Raynald, "When you can fit through the doorway you can leave."
>
> King Edward then instructed his servants to bring massive platters of meat and other delicacies and daily place them on the table in Raynald's round dungeon room. The servants also filled the table with various kinds of pies and pastries. Many people accused Edward of being cruel, but he would respond, "My brother is not a prisoner. He can leave when he chooses to."
>
> Now for the rest of the story: Raynald remained in that same room, a prisoner of his own appetite, for more than ten years. He wasn't released until later after Edward died in battle. By then his own health was so far gone that he died within a year—not because he had no choice, but because he would not use his power to choose what was best for his life.[3]

This graphic story illustrates that knowledge alone about relief from a problem is not enough. You must act on your knowledge to change your circumstances. It is possible to feel bad about a situation, but not bad enough to change.

You have gained knowledge about what causes headaches. You have also gained knowledge about how to prevent or reduce the severity of headaches. Now the question arises, "Do you want to stay in the headache dungeon, or do you want to get out?"

The doorway to the headache dungeon is open. You can escape when:

- Stress is reduced.
- Diet is restructured.
- Exercise begins.
- Schedules are modified.
- Adrenaline is controlled.
- Allergies are acknowledged.
- Medications are adjusted.
- Environment is altered.
- Thinking changes.
- Emotional problems are addressed.
- Relationships are healed.

This is not to say that the way out of the dungeon is easy. It is not. But the end result is very freeing. It causes one to rejoice. It also encourages one to share the good news of escape with others who may still be trapped and seeing no way out. There is hope, and it is all at your fingertips.

# Notes

### *Chapter 1*
### *The High Cost of Headaches*

1. Bob Phillips, *Phillips Awesome Collection of Quips and Quotes* (Eugene, OR: Harvest House Publishers, 2001).

2. Zuzana and Francis Bic, *No More Headaches No More Migraines* (New York, NY: Avery, 1999), 17.

3. David Buchholz, *Heal Your Headache* (New York, NY: Workman Publishing, 2002), 1.

4. Lynne Constantine and Suzanne Scott, *Migraine: The Complete Guide* (N.p.: Delta, 1994), 17.

5. Dr. Frank Minirth, *The Headache Book* (Nashville, TN: Thomas Nelson Publishers, 1994), 2.

6. Oliver Sacks, *Migraine* (Los Angeles, CA: University of California Press, 1992), 1.

7. *World Book Encyclopedia*, vol. 21 (Chicago, IL: Field Enterprises Educational Corporation, 1976), s.v. "Washington, George."

### *Chapter 2*
### *Theories About Headaches*

1. Phillips, *Phillips Awesome Collection of Quips and Quotes.*

2. Adapted from Roger Cady and Kathleen Farmer, *Headache Free* (New York, NY: Bantam Books, 1996), 26.

### *Chapter 3*
### *Various Types of Headaches*

1. Constantine and Scott, *Migraine: The Complete Guide*, 69.

2. Ibid., 69–70.

### *Chapter 4*
### *Physical Causes of Headaches*

1. Bob Phillips, *Great Thoughts and Funny Sayings* (Wheaton, IL: Tyndale House Publishers, 1993).

2. Mark W. Green and Leah M. Green, *Managing Your Headaches* (New York, NY: Springer-Verlag, 2001), 42.

### *Chapter 5*
### *Environmental Causes of Headaches*

1. Information regarding nitroglycerin was adapted from the following sources: "Nitroglycerin," Britannica Guide to the Nobel Prizes, http://www.britannica.com/nobel/micro/426_77.html (accessed December 1, 2004); "Nitrogylcerin," MedicineNet.com, http://www.medicinenet.com/nitroglycerin/article.htm, (accessed December 1, 2004).

### *Chapter 6*
### *Emotional Causes of Headaches*

1. Phillips, *Phillips Awesome Collection of Quips and Quotes.*

### *Chapter 7*
### *Food Causes of Headaches*

1. Jonathan Swift, *Prose Works of Jonathan Swift,* (N.p.: AMS Press, 1940).

2. Charles B. Inlander and Porter Shimer, *Headaches—47 Ways to Stop the Pain* (New York, NY: Walker and Company, 1995), 24.

3. Neil Nedley, *Proof Positive—How to Reliably Combat Disease and Achieve Optimal Health Through Nutrition and Lifestyle* (Ardmore, OK: Neil Nedley, 1998), 187.

4. Ibid., 30–33.

### *Chapter 8*
### *Headache Discovery Guide*

1. Phillips, *Phillips Awesome Collection of Quips and Quotes.*

2. David E. Bresler, *Free Yourself From Pain* (New York, NY: Simon and Schuster, 1979), 244–250.

3. T. H. Holmes and R. H. Rahe, "The Social Readjustment Rating Scale," *Journal of Psychosomatic Research* 2 (1967): 213–218. Used by permission of Elsevier Science Publications.

### *Chapter 9*
### *Drug-Free Strategies for Headache Relief*

1. Phillips, *Phillips Awesome Collection of Quips and Quotes,* 201.

### *Chapter 10*
### *Physical Strategies for Headache Relief*

1. Phillips, *Phillips Awesome Collection of Quips and Quotes.*

2. Pete E. Egoscue, *Pain Free* (New York, NY: Bantam Books, 1998), 198.

3. Tim LaHaye and Bob Phillips, *Anger Is a Choice* (Grand Rapids, MI: Zondervan Publishing House, 1982), 35–38.

4. Bresler, *Free Yourself From Pain*, 167–168.

5. Ibid., 201.

6. Adapted from Daniel Girdano, et al., *Controlling Stress and Tension* (Englewood Cliffs, NJ: Prentice-Hall, Inc., 1979), 227–229.

7. Robert S. Ivker and Todd Nelson, *Headache Survival* (New York, NY: Jeremy P. Tarcher, 2002).

8. Bresler, *Free Yourself From Pain*, 148–150.

### *Chapter 11*
### *Diet and Medical Strategies for Headache Relief*

1. Phillips, *Phillips Awesome Collection of Quips and Quotes.*

2. The complied list is from Zuzana and L. Francis Bic, *No More Headaches No More Migraines*, 115–120, and Paula Maas and Deborah Mitchel, *Guide to Headache Relief* (New York, NY: A Lynn Sonberg book, 1997), 179–185.

### *Chapter 12*
### *Psychological and Spiritual Strategies for Headache Relief*

1. Phillips, *Phillips Awesome Collection of Quips and Quotes.*

2. Sacks, *Migraine*, xvii–xviii.

3. Phillips, *Phillips Awesome Collection of Quips and Quotes.*

4. Ibid.

5. Phillips, *Great Thoughts and Funny Sayings*, 18.

6. Phillips, *Phillips Awesome Collection of Quips and Quotes.*

### *Chapter 13*
### *Miscellaneous Strategies for Headache Relief*

1. Phillips, *Phillips Awesome Collection of Quips and Quotes.*

2. Cady and Farmer, *Headache Free*, 39–41.

3. John Mansfield, *Migraine: The Drug-Free Solution* (Rochester, VT: Thorsons Publishers, Inc., 1987), 67–68.

***Conclusion***

1. Bob Phillips, *The Star-Spangled Quote Book* (Eugene, OR: Harvest House Publishers, 1997), 59.

2. Phillips, *Phillips Awesome Collection of Quips and Quotes.*

3. Bob Phillips, *Getting Off the Emotional Roller Coaster* (Eugene, OR: Harvest House Publishers, 2001), 39–40.

# Scripture Index

**DESPAIR**
Exodus 14:1–14
Psalm 40

**DIFFICULTIES**
Romans 8:28
2 Corinthians 4:17
Hebrews 12:7–11
Revelation 3:19

**DISAPPOINTMENT**
Psalms 43:5; 55:22; 126:6
John 14:27
2 Corinthians 4:8–17

**DISCOURAGEMENT**
Joshua 1:9
Psalm 27:14
Colossians 1:5
1 Peter 1:3–9
1 John 5:14

**DISCERNMENT**
Matthew 7:1–12
1 Corinthians 2:12–16
Hebrews 5:13–14
James 1:2–8

**DISHONESTY**
Leviticus 19:35–36
Proverbs 20:10, 14, 17, 23
Luke 16:1–12

**DISOBEDIENCE**
Genesis 3
1 Chronicles 13

**DIVORCE AND REMARRIAGE**
Malachi 2:15–16
Matthew 19:8–9
1 Corinthians 7:10–15

**DRINKING**
Proverbs 23:29–35
Ephesians 5:15–20

**ENCOURAGEMENT**
1 Thessalonians 5
1 Peter 1:1–13

**ENTHUSIASM**
Colossians 3:23–25

**ENVY**
Deuteronomy 5:21
Numbers 12:1–10

**ETERNAL LIFE**
Luke 18:18–30
John 3:1–21; 6:60–71; 17
1 John 5:1–13

**FAULTS**
Hosea 4:4–6
Matthew 7:1–5
Ephesians 4:1–3

**FEAR**
Joshua 1
Psalms 27:1; 56:11; 91:1–6; 121
Proverbs 29:25

**FOOLISHNESS**
Psalm 14
Proverbs 9
1 Corinthians 2:6–16

**FORGIVENESS**
Psalm 51
Matthew 6:5–15; 18:21–35
1 John 1

**FRIENDSHIP**
Proverbs 17:9, 17; 22:24–27; 27:6, 9–10
John 15:1–17

**FRUSTRATION**
Ephesians 6:1–4

**GAMBLING**
Proverbs 15:16; 23:4–5
Luke 12:15
1 Timothy 6:9

**GENTLENESS**
2 Timothy 2:24–26
James 3:17–18

**GOSSIP**
Exodus 23:1–9
Proverbs 25:18–28
2 Thessalonians 3:6–15

**GREED**
James 4:13–17
1 John 2:15–17

**RELATIONSHIPS**
2 Corinthians 6:14–18
Ephesians 2:11–22

**RESENTMENT**
Hebrews 12:1–15

**REVENGE**
Romans 12:17–21

**SELF-CENTEREDNESS**
Mark 8:31–38
1 Peter 1:14–25

**SELFISHNESS**
Mark 8:31–38
Romans 12
James 4:1–10

**SEX**
Proverbs 5:15–21
1 Corinthians 7:1–11
1 Thessalonians 4:1–8

**SICKNESS**
Psalms 41:3; 103:3
Matthew 4:23–25
John 11:4
James 5:13–15

**SIN**
Isaiah 53:5–6; 59:1–2
John 8:34
Romans 3:23; 6:23
Galatians 6:7–8

**STRESS**
Romans 5:1–5
Philippians 4:4–9

**SUFFERING**
Romans 8:18
2 Corinthians 1:5
Philippians 3:10
2 Timothy 2:12
James 1:2–8
1 Peter 1:6–7

**SUICIDE**
Job 14:5
Romans 14:7
1 Corinthians 6:19–20
James 4:7

**TEMPTATION**
Psalm 94:17–18
Proverbs 28:13
1 Corinthians 10:12–13
Hebrews 4:14–16
James 1:2–14

**TERMINAL ILLNESS**
Jeremiah 29:11
2 Corinthians 12:9
1 Thessalonians 5:18
2 Timothy 2:10–11

**THANKFULNESS**
Psalm 92
Romans 1:21
Ephesians 5:20

**WAITING**
Psalms 27; 40:14
Matthew 24:32–51

**WEAKNESS**
2 Corinthians 12:1–10
1 John 3:1–11

**WILL OF GOD**
Psalms 37:4; 91:1–2
Proverbs 3:5–6; 4:26
Romans 14:5
Galatians 6:4
Ephesians 5:15–21
Philippians 2:12–13
1 Thessalonians 4:3
1 Peter 3:17

**WISDOM**
Psalm 119:97–112
Proverbs 1:1–7
Ecclesiastes 8:1–8
Luke 2:21–40
James 1:2–8

**WORRY**
Psalm 37:1–11
Matthew 6:25–34
Philippians 4:4–9

# Topical Index

# Bibliography


Bic, Zuzana, and L. Francis Bic. *No More Headaches—No More Migraines.* New York, NY: Avery, 1999.

Biermann, June, and Barbara Toohey. *The Woman's Holistic Headache Relief Book.* New York, NY: Tarcher Publishers.

Bresler, David E. *Free Yourself From Pain.* New York, NY: Simon and Schuster, 1979.

Buchholz, David, and Stephen G. Reich. *Heal Your Headache: The 1-2-3 Program for Taking Charge of Your Pain.* New York, NY: Workman Publishing, 2002.

Cady, Roger, and Kathleen Farmer. *Headache Free.* New York, NY: Bantam Books, 1996.

Constantine, Lynne M., and Suzanne Scott. *Migraine: The Complete Guide.* New York, NY: Dell Publishing, 1994.

Culligan, Matthew J., and Keith Sedlacek. *How to Avoid Stress Before It Kills You.* New York, NY: Gramercy Publishing, 1980.

Egoscue, Pete. *Pain Free: A Revolutionary Method for Stopping Chronic Pain.* New York, NY: Bantam Books, 1998.

Faelten, Sharon. *No More Headaches.* Emmaus, PA: Rodale Press, 1982.

Gillespie, Peggy Roggenbuck, and Lynn Bechtel. *Less Stress in Thirty Days.* New York, NY: A Plume Book, 1986.

Girdano, Daniel, and George Everly. *Controlling Stress and Tension: A Holistic Approach.* Englewood Cliffs, NJ: Prentice-Hall, Inc., 1979.

Green, Mark W., and Leah M. Green. *Managing Your Headaches.* New York, NY: Springer-Verlag, 2001.

Harpe, Shideler. *Headaches: Causes and Cures.* Chicago, IL: Budlong Press, 1979.

Hart, Archibald D. *Adrenaline and Stress.* Dallas, TX: Word Publishing, 1991.

Inlander, Charles B., and Porter Shimer. *Headaches: 47 Ways to Stop the Pain.* New York, NY: Walker and Company, 1995.

Ivker, Robert S. and Todd Nelson. *Headache Survival.* New York, NY: Jeremy P. Tarcher/Putnam, 2002.

Krames, Lawrence A. *The Back Owners Manual.* Los Angeles, CA: Price/Stern/Sloan, 1979.

Kurland, Howard D. *Quick Headache Relief Without Drugs.* New York, NY: William Morrow & Company, Inc., 1977.

LaHaye, Tim and Bob Phillips. *Anger Is a Choice.* Grand Rapids, MI: Zondervan Publishing House, 1982.

MacLennan, Doug. *How to Keep Fit at Your Desk.* Los Angeles, CA: Price/Stern/Sloan, 1980.

Mansfield, John. *Migraine: The Drug-Free Solution.* Rochester, VT: Thorsons Publishers, Inc., 1987.

Maas, Paula, and Deborah Mitchel. *Guide to Headache Relief.* New York, NY: A Lynn Sonberg Book, 1997.

Melzack, Ronald. *The Puzzle of Pain.* New York, NY: Basic Books, 1973.

Miller, Emmett E. *Feeling Good: How to Stay Healthy.* Englewood Cliffs, NJ: Prentice-Hall, Inc., 1978.

Miller, Joan. *Headaches: The Answer Book.* Old Tappan, NJ: Fleming H. Revell Company, 1983.

Minirth, Frank. *The Headache Book.* Nashville, TN: Thomas Nelson Publishers, 1994.

Morehouse, Laurence E. and Leonard Gross. *Total Fitness in 30 Minutes a Week.* New York, NY: Pocket Books, 1975.

Narramore, Clyde M. *How to Handle Pressure.* Wheaton, IL: Coverdale House, 1975.

Nedley, Neil. *Proof Positive: How to Reliably Combat Disease and Achieve Optimal Health Through Nutrition and Lifestyle.* Ardmore, OK: Neil Nedley, 1998.

Phillips, Bob. *Getting Off the Emotional Roller Coaster.* Eugene, OR: Harvest House Publishers, 2001.

———. *Great Thoughts and Funny Sayings.* Wheaton, IL: Tyndale House Publishers, 1993.

———. *Phillips Awesome Collections of Quips and Quotes.* Eugene, OR: Harvest House Publishers, 2001.

———. *The All-American Quote Book.* Eugene, OR: Harvest House Publishers, 1995.

———. *The Star-Spangled Quote Book.* Eugene, OR: Harvest House Publishers, 1997.

———. *Values and Virtues.* Sisters, OR: Questar Publishers, 1997.

Sacks, Oliver. *Migraine*. Los Angeles, CA: University of California Press, 1992.

Selye, Hans. *Stress Without Distress*. New York, NY: A Signet Book, 1974.

Sehnert, Keith W. *Stress/Unstress*. Minneapolis, MN: Augsburg Publishing House, 1981.

Tubesing, Donald. *Kicking Your Stress Habits*. New York, NY: A Signet Book, 1981

Tubesing, Nancy Loving, and Donald A. Tubesing. *Structured Exercises in Stress Management*. Duluth, MN: Whole Person Press, 1983.

**BOOKS WRITTEN BY BOB PHILLIPS**

may be purchased through:

FAMILY SERVICES

P. O. Box 9363

Fresno, CA 93792

*[Send a self-addressed stamped envelope for a list of books.]*

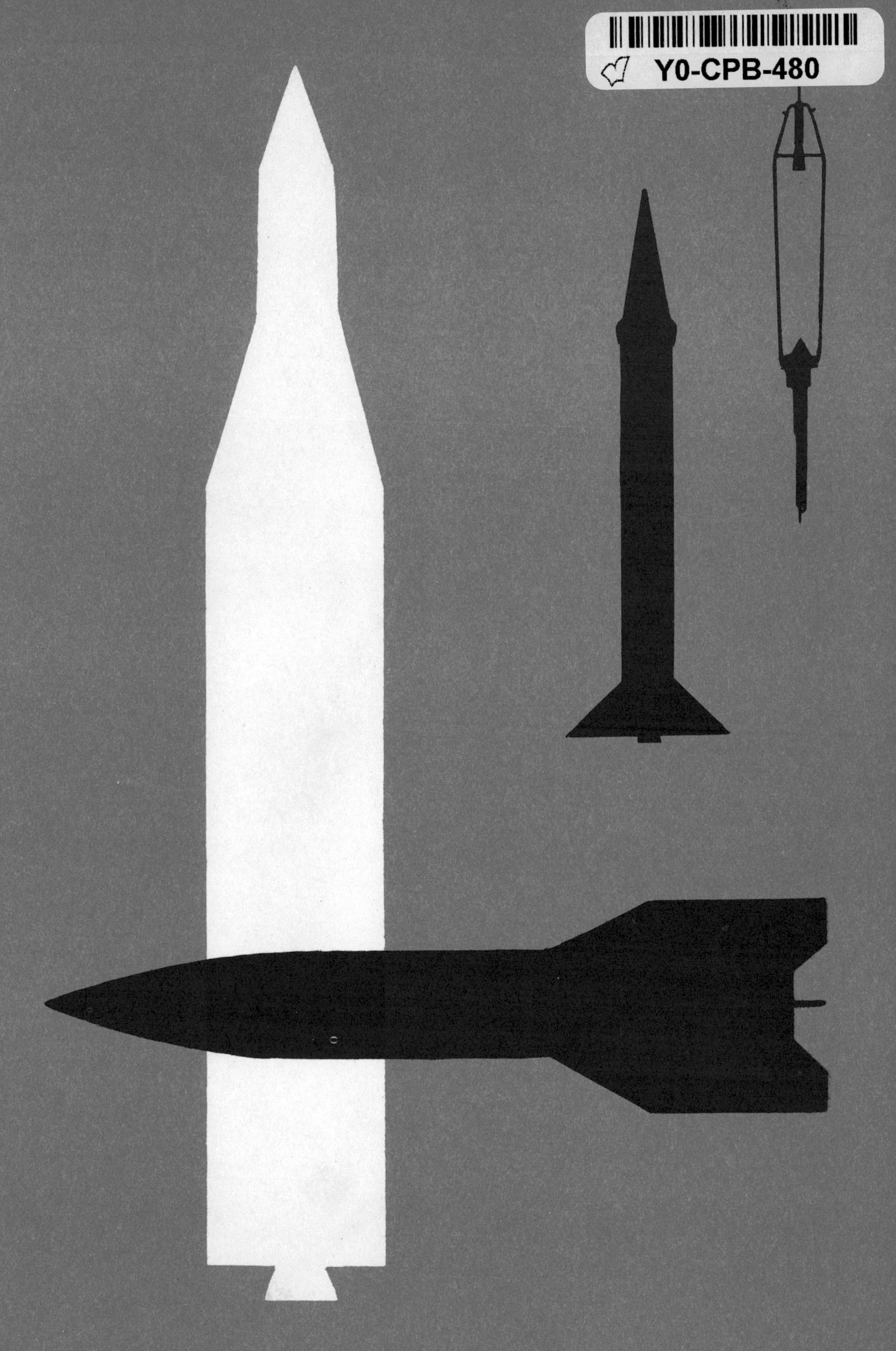

# ROCKETS INTO SPACE

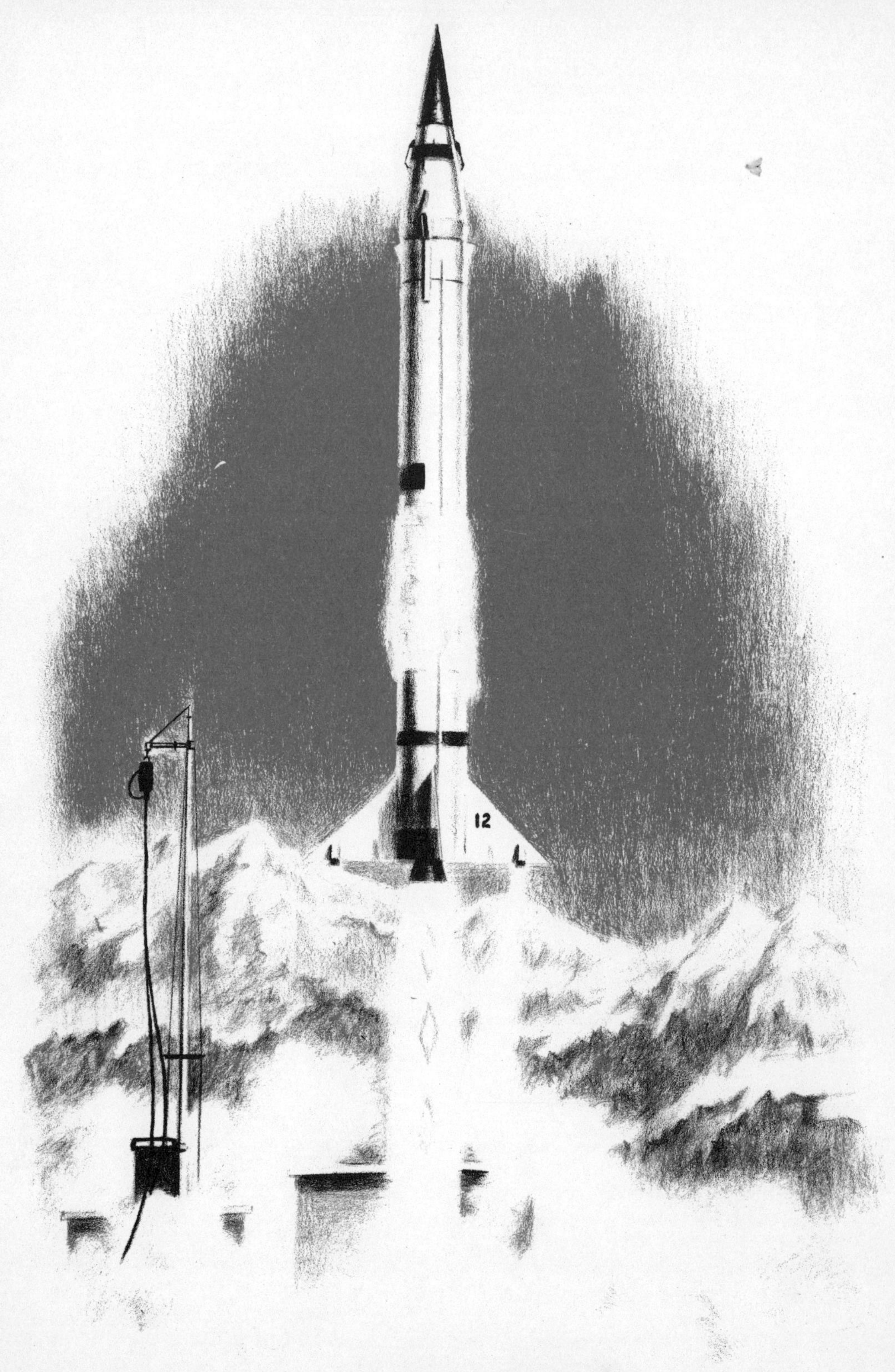

# ROCKETS INTO SPACE

*by Alexander L. Crosby and Nancy Larrick*

ILLUSTRATED BY DENNY McMAINS

RANDOM HOUSE · NEW YORK

The authors and the artist are grateful to the following for assistance in the preparation of this book: John Newbauer, associate editor of *Astronautics;* Bernard Maggin, of the National Aeronautics and Space Administration; G. Edward Pendray, founding member of the American Rocket Society; Convair Division of the General Dynamics Corporation; and the New York offices of the Departments of Information, U.S. Army and U.S. Air Force.

 Published in New York by Random House, Inc., and simultaneously in Toronto, Canada, by Random House of Canada, Limited.

Library of Congress Catalog Card Number: 59-12360

Manufactured in the United States of America

# CONTENTS

# ROCKETS INTO SPACE

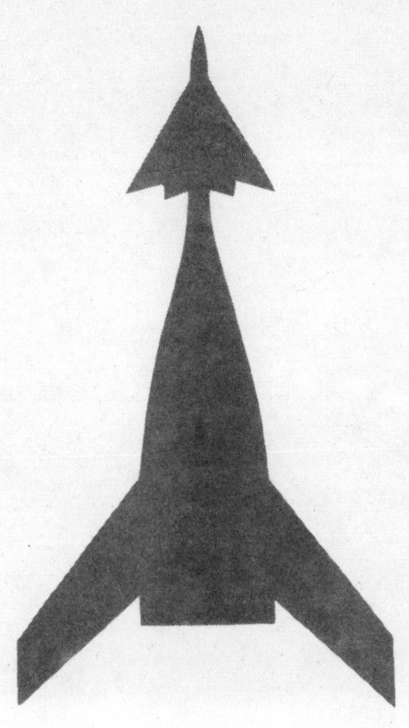

# 1
# BEYOND THIS WORLD

How would it feel to stand on the moon?

In a few years, men in space suits will walk on the moon. They will look at the sun and stars shining in a black sky. They will see the bluish earth, four times as big as the moon looks to us.

Rocket ships will take men to the moon. These

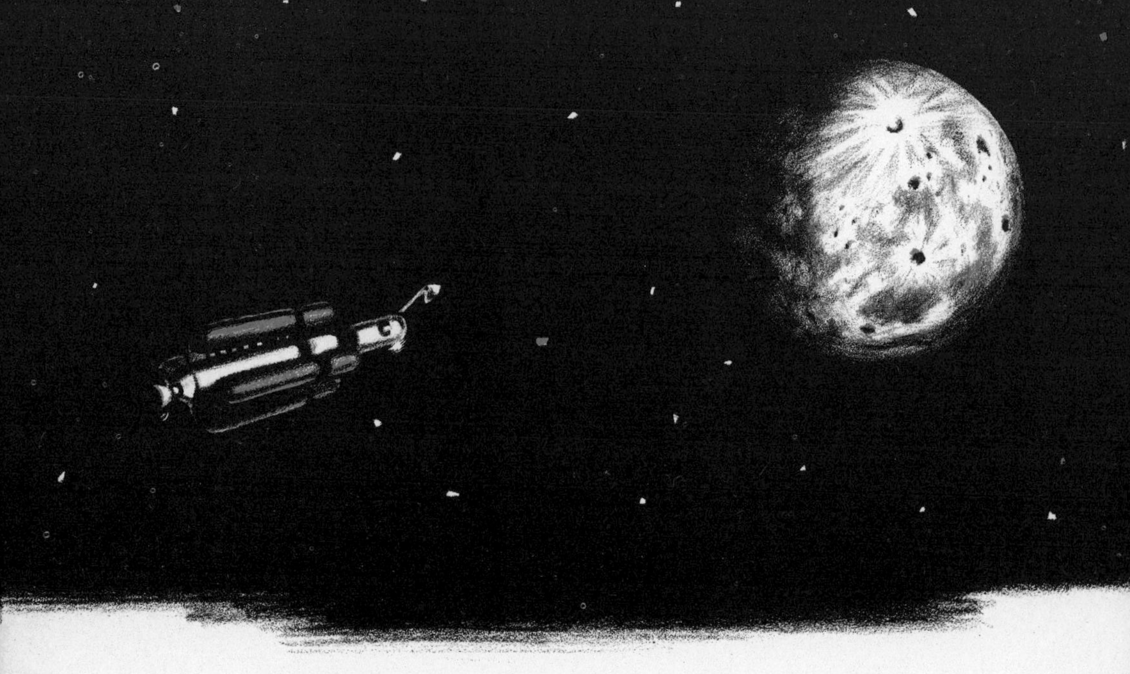

*Rocket ships will take men to the moon.*

space travelers will find answers to many secrets of the universe.

Long ago people believed the earth was the center of the whole universe. They thought the earth was bigger than the sun.

Then people learned that the earth is very tiny. It is like one grain of sand on a beach that stretches out of sight. Our sun is only one of millions and millions of suns.

These suns are called stars. You can see some of

them at night. If you had a telescope, you could see many more.

It's hard to imagine how far away the stars are. Suppose you watch an airplane beacon on a mountain several miles away. The flash of light reaches you right away.

The sun is so far away that its light takes eight minutes to reach the earth. Light from the nearest star travels four years before it can be seen on earth. Some stars take millions of years to send their light to us.

The universe is bigger than anyone can imagine. Scientists are not sure whether it ends anywhere. Maybe it just keeps stretching into space forever and ever.

The earth is one of nine planets that move around the sun. Some are bigger than the earth, and some are smaller. The largest is Jupiter. This planet is more than a thousand times bigger than the earth.

Venus is the brightest planet. You can often

PLUTO

NEPTUNE

URANUS

THE SUN AND ITS NINE PLANETS

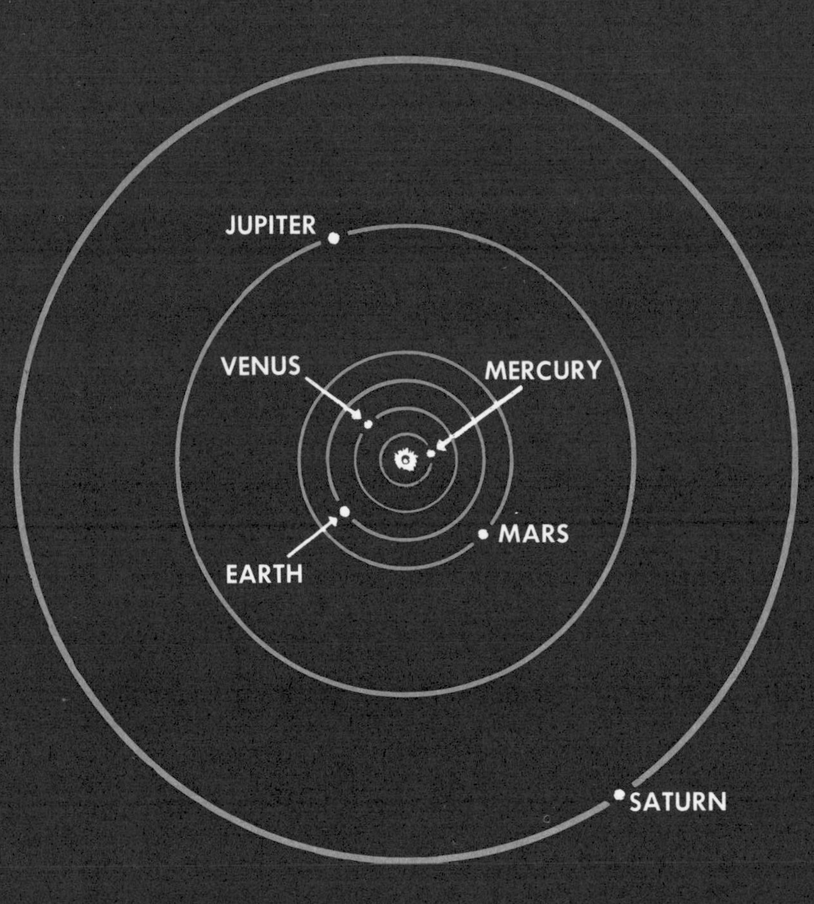
JUPITER
VENUS
MERCURY
EARTH
MARS
SATURN

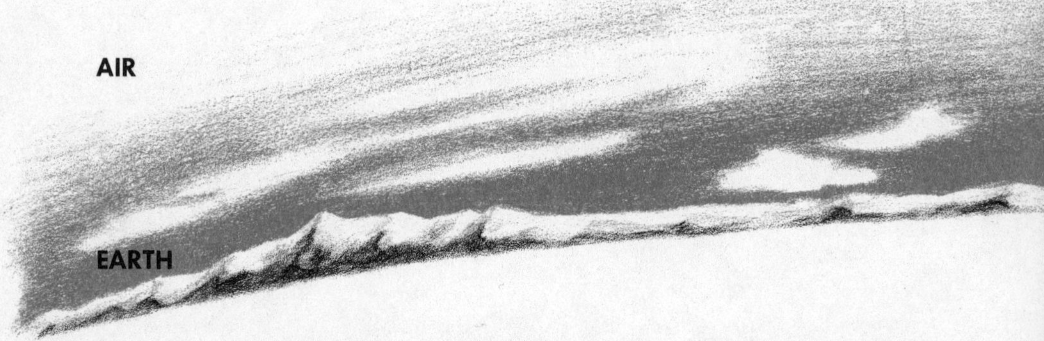


*The air is thickest near the earth's surface.*

see it in the evening sky. If you get up very early, you can see Venus before sunrise.

Mars is called the red planet because, as you may know, it looks red.

Most of the planets have satellites. These are smaller bodies that circle around the planet. The earth has only one natural satellite: the moon.

The sun and the stars are huge balls of hot gases. The earth and some other planets are made of rock and other minerals. The moon is probably solid.

Pictures of the planets have been made with powerful telescopes. But the best pictures have

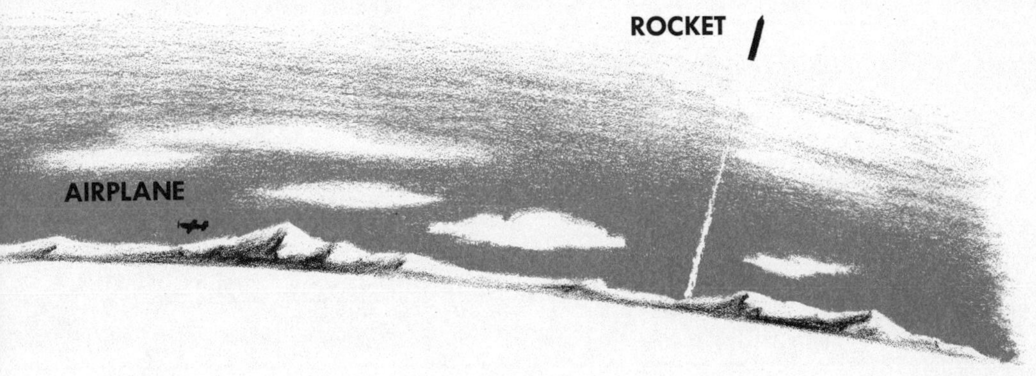


*Twenty miles up there is almost no air.*

been taken of the moon. That's because the moon is much closer than the planets.

For thousands of years, men have wondered about the moon and the planets. What made the big craters on the moon? Are there any living creatures on the planets? Do plants grow on Mars?

The only way to find out is by going to the moon and to the planets.

The earth has a blanket of air around it. At sea level the air is thickest. As we go higher, the air gets thinner. Twenty miles up, there is practically no air. That is the beginning of space.

We can't explore space with an airplane, because an airplane needs air. There is no air in outer space.

But there is a way to get to the moon and even to the distant planets. That is by rocket ship. We are learning to build rockets that will take us into space.

Rockets are not a new invention. But the rockets we are building today go farther and faster than any rockets in history.

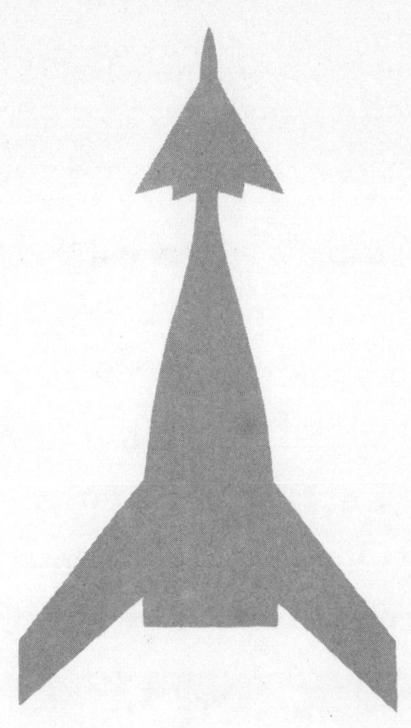

# 2

# HOW A ROCKET WORKS

More than a thousand years ago, the Chinese made a great discovery. They mixed some chemical powders together. When fire touched the powders, they blew up.

This mixture was gunpowder.

We don't know what happened to the first man

who set fire to gunpowder. He may have blown up, too.

The Chinese soon learned how to make a big noise with a teaspoonful of gunpowder. They wrapped the powder very tightly in a small roll of paper and closed both ends.

In one end, they left a tiny hole for a fuse. The fuse was a twist of thin paper with a few grains of powder inside.

There were no matches in those days. Sparks were made by striking a piece of iron against a very hard stone called flint. The Chinese lit the fuse by making sparks with iron and flint.

The fuse sputtered as it burned. When the fire reached the gunpowder inside, the whole tube blew up with a bang.

This was a firecracker.

Why does a firecracker blow up? Because the gunpowder inside burns very fast. It burns faster than paper or even oil. As it burns, it makes hot gases that push in all directions.

The gases push against the paper walls of the tube,

trying to escape. They press so hard they blow the tube into bits with a loud bang.

The Chinese found many ways to use firecrackers. They exploded them on holidays. The noise was supposed to scare away evil spirits.

Sometimes people in Chinese towns were attacked by warriors from the mountains. The war-

*The Chinese scared enemies with firecrackers.*

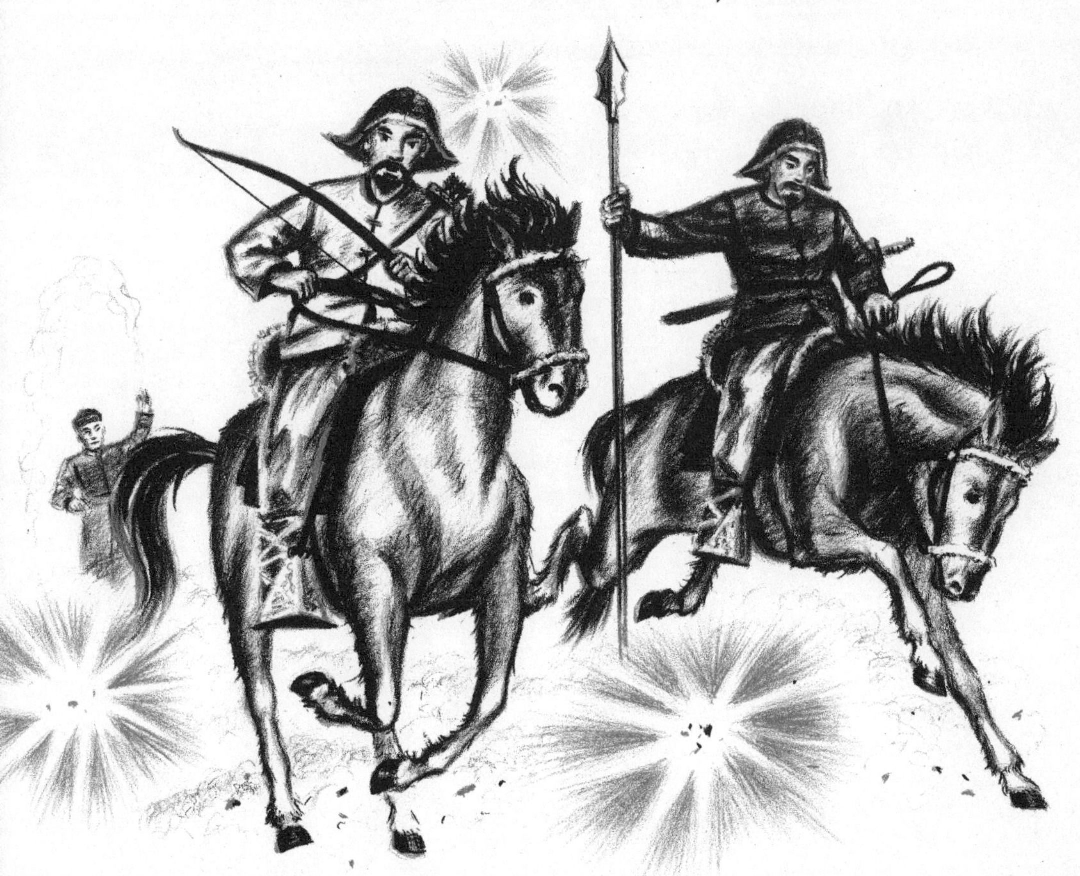

riors rode horses and carried spears and swords. There were no guns then.

The town people threw firecrackers at their enemies. The firecrackers made the horses run away. The warriors were scared, too.

A firecracker doesn't go far when a man throws it. The Chinese wanted their firecrackers to go much farther. So they tried something different.

They packed gunpowder into a heavy paper tube. It was about as thick as a broomstick and as long as your hand.

They tied the tube to a thin stick so that it would go through the air like an arrow. Then they put a spark to the powder at the bottom of the tube. The tube and stick shot into the air with a *whoosh!*

This was the first rocket.

Why didn't it blow up like a firecracker? It didn't blow up because the bottom of the tube was left open. The hot gases could escape as the powder burned.

As the burning gases rushed backward, they

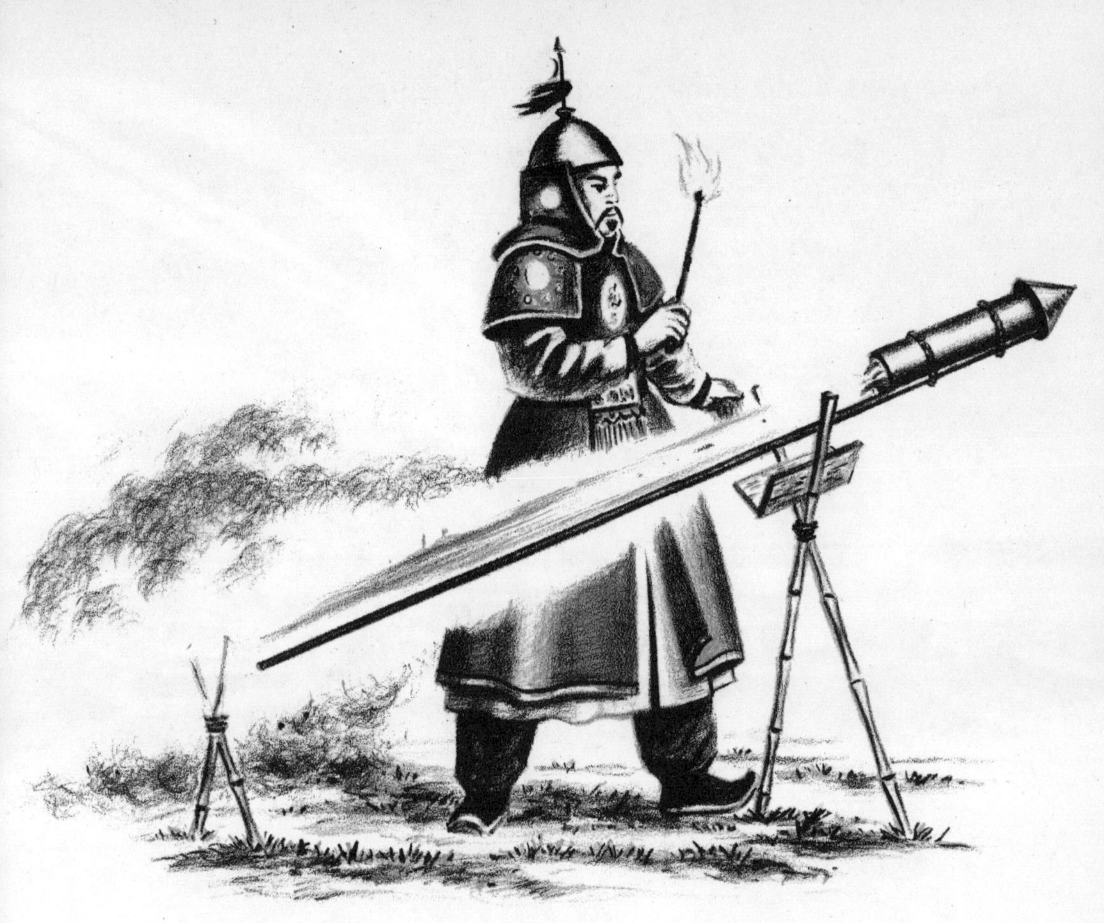

*The Chinese learned to improve their early rockets.*

pushed the rocket forward. That is why a rocket zooms through the air.

You can see how this works if you watch a man

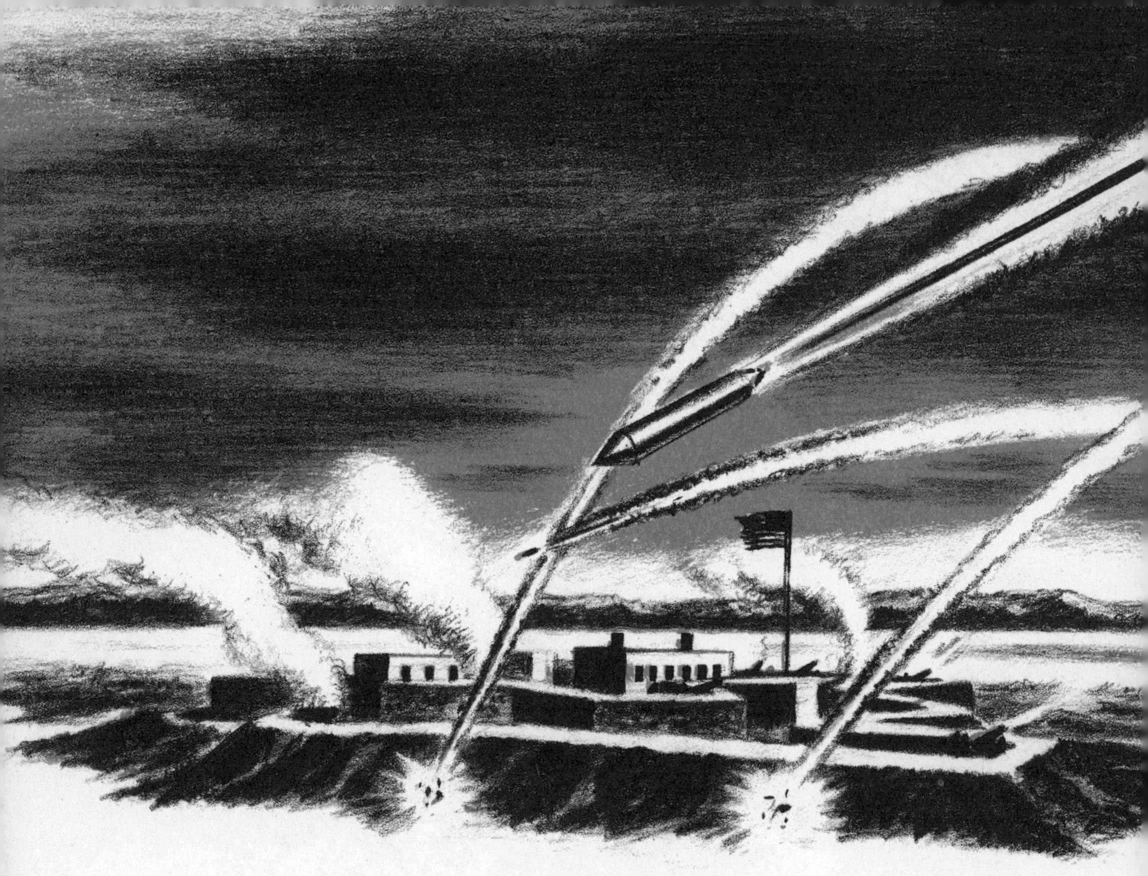

*In the War of 1812 the British fired rockets at Americans.*

fire a rifle. The gun kicks back against his shoulder as the bullet shoots ahead.

The same kind of kick makes a rocket go.

The Chinese soon learned how to make better rockets. They put a pointed cone on the front end of the tube. This streamlined the rocket. Streamlining made it go faster and straighter.

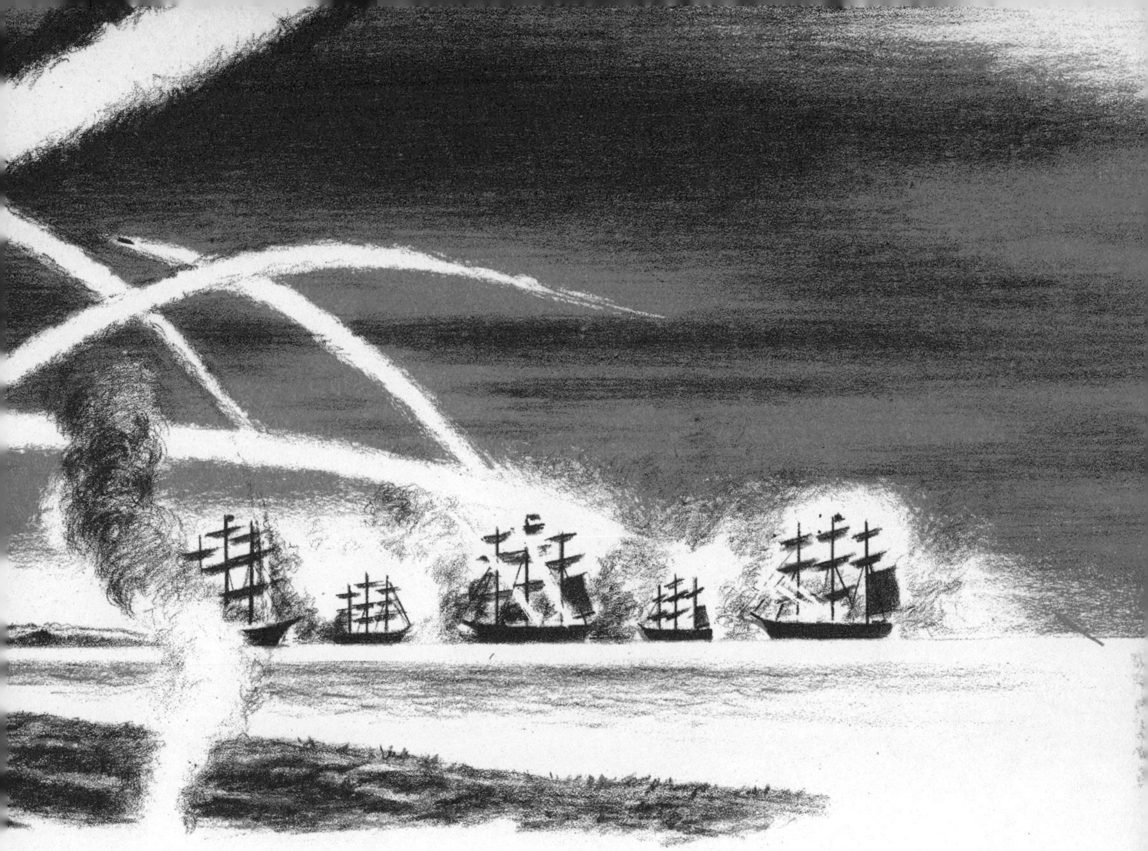

*British ships could be seen in the "rockets' red glare."*

The secret of the rocket was finally learned by other countries. The armies of Europe used a great many rockets. Extra gunpowder was fastened inside the nose of the rocket. The gunpowder exploded when the rocket landed among enemy soldiers.

Towns were set on fire by rockets that fell on

roofs. The British used rockets against the Americans in the War of 1812. "The Star-Spangled Banner" mentions "the rockets' red glare."

Rockets went out of fashion when big guns were made more accurate. The rockets of the last century were hit-or-miss weapons—mostly miss.

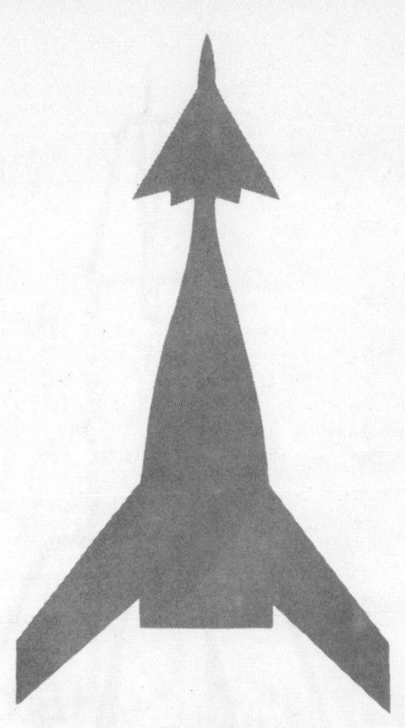

# 3

# PROFESSOR GODDARD'S ROCKET

The year 1926 is famous in the history of rockets. It was made famous by an American professor, Robert Hutchins Goddard. He was curious about space, above the earth's air blanket. He thought he could find some answers by building a new kind of rocket.

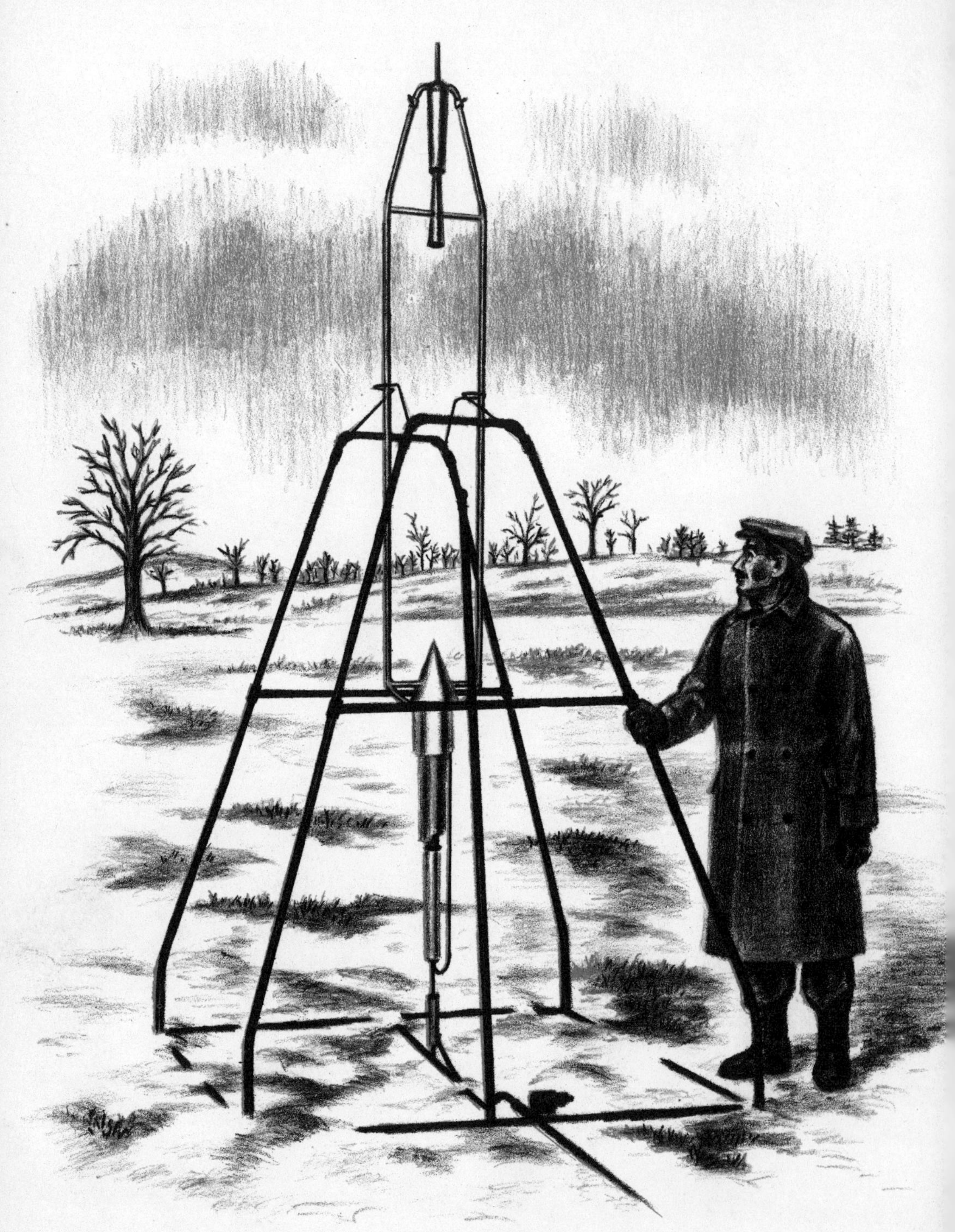

*Goddard fired the first liquid-fuel rocket.*

He did not use gunpowder. He used two liquids that would burn at a terrific rate. One was gasoline. The other was liquid oxygen. Oxygen makes anything burn very fast.

Professor Goddard built a rocket that was taller than a man. He took it to his aunt's farm at Auburn, Massachusetts, on March 16, 1926. He lit the fuel.

The rocket whizzed into the air with a tremendous roar. It flew a little less than a city block before it came down in the snow.

This was the first time a rocket had ever gone up without gunpowder.

The gasoline mixture was better than gunpowder. It had more power.

Professor Goddard had discovered the key to modern rockets. His first rocket flight was probably as important as the first airplane flight of the Wright brothers.

But he didn't get a letter from the President or a medal from Congress. The only officials who came to see him were a squad of angry cops. They came in a hurry when one of his rockets flew with a terrific noise. People were frightened for miles around.

A few other scientists began to experiment with liquid-fuel rockets. They used to pick lonely beaches and empty fields for tests. But even a small rocket made such a big noise that people nearby were alarmed.

G. Edward Pendray, one of the pioneers, remembers those days.

"As soon as we launched our rocket, we took off, too," he says. "We knew the cops would be there within half an hour."

Except for the scientists, nobody imagined that rockets would ever carry passengers. People said it was ridiculous to talk about going to the moon by rocket.

The rocket pioneers had very little money for their experiments. If they had been given real help, we might be making trips to the moon today.

In World War II the Germans built a rocket as tall as a four-story building. This was called the V-2. Like Professor Goddard's rocket, it burned liquid fuel and flew very fast.

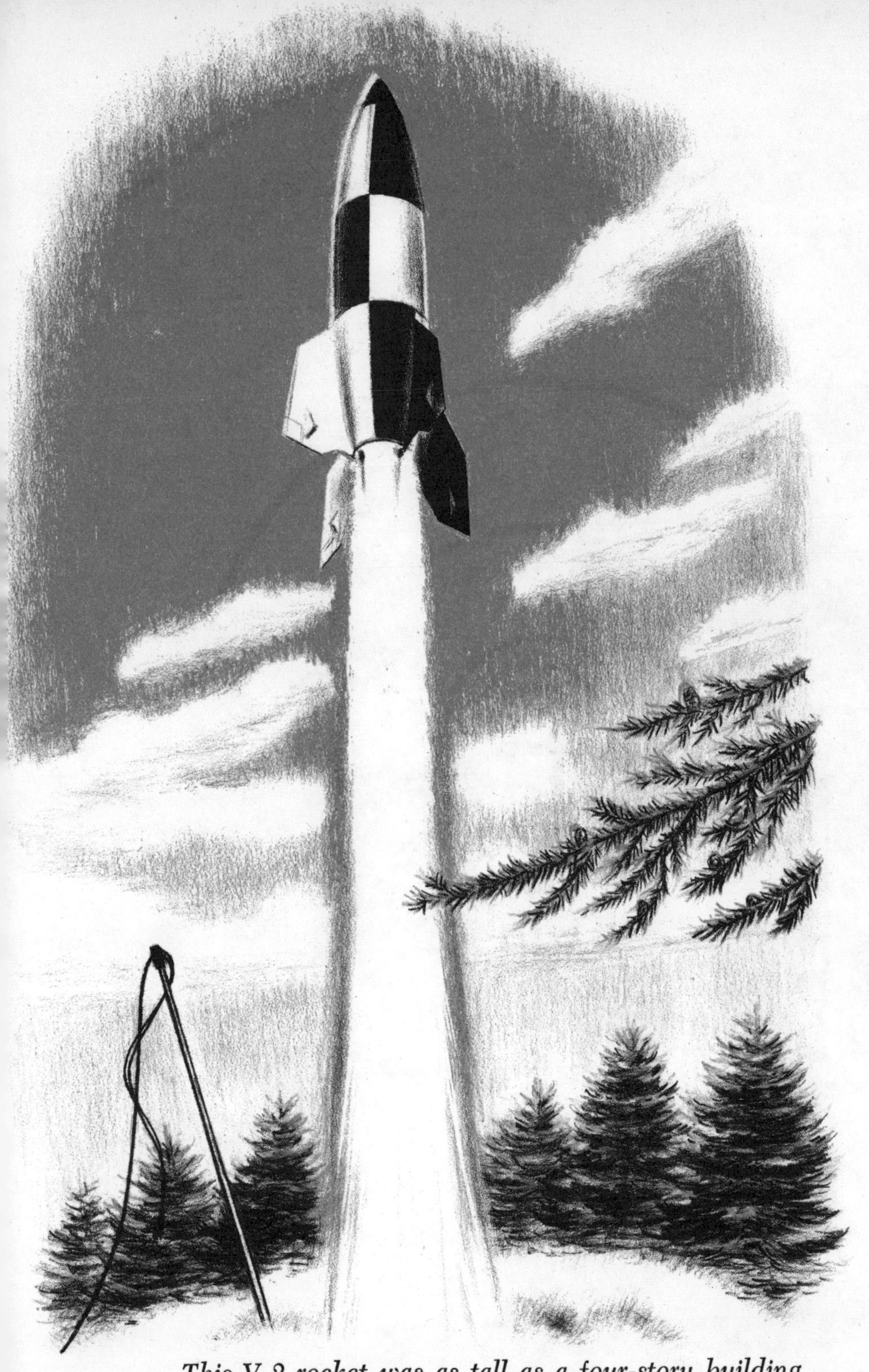

*This V-2 rocket was as tall as a four-story building.*

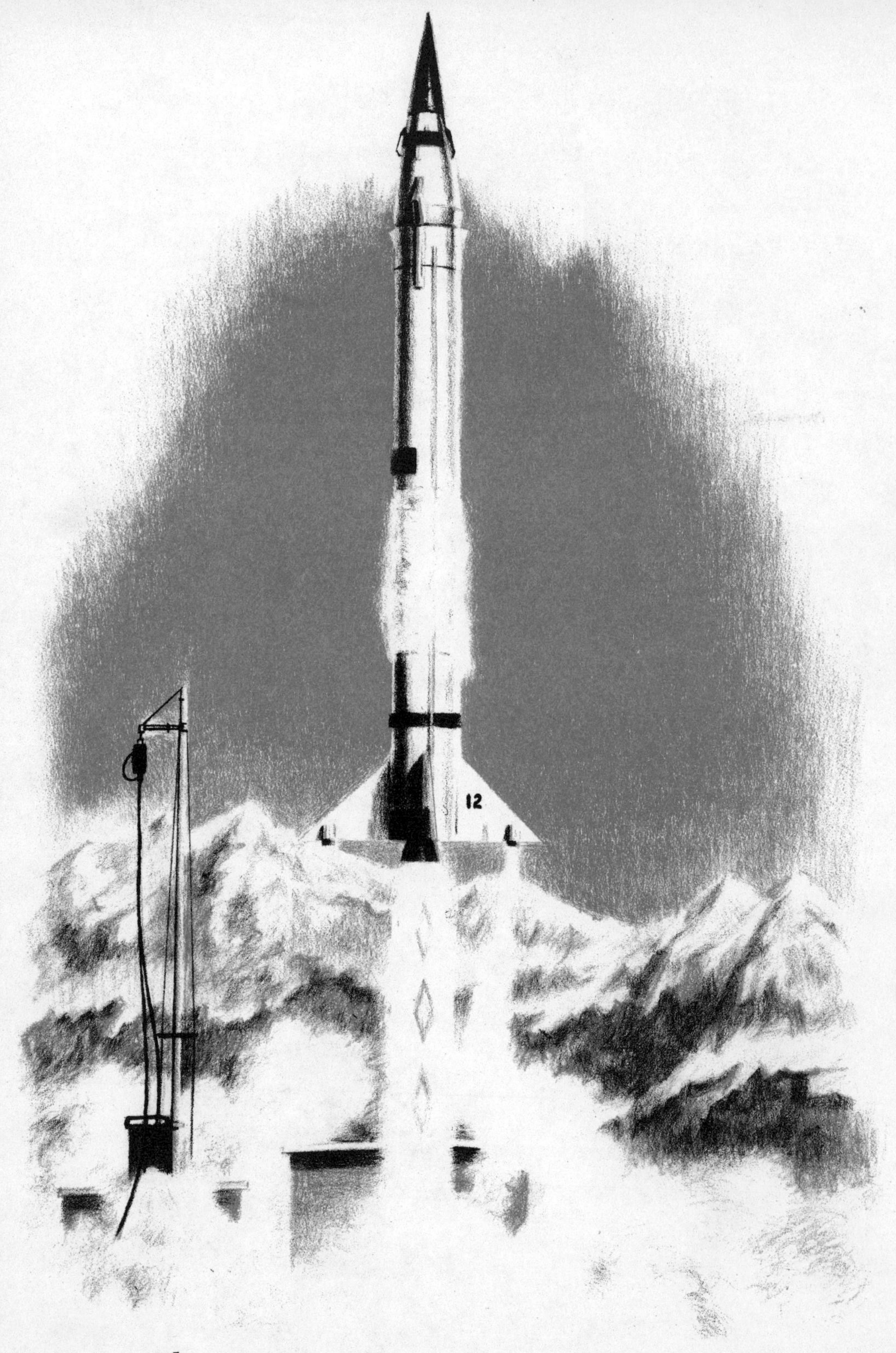


*The American Viking rocket was five stories tall.*

The Germans fired more than 1,000 of these big rockets at the city of London. Many people were killed.

American soldiers captured some of these German rockets at the end of the war. The rockets were sent back to the United States. Scientists took them apart to see how they were made.

Soon we were building our own giant rockets. We sent them many miles up into the sky. The rockets went much farther than man has ever gone in a balloon or airplane.

Each rocket carried scientific instruments. The instruments told how hot or cold the sky was. They gave new facts about the cosmic rays in outer space.

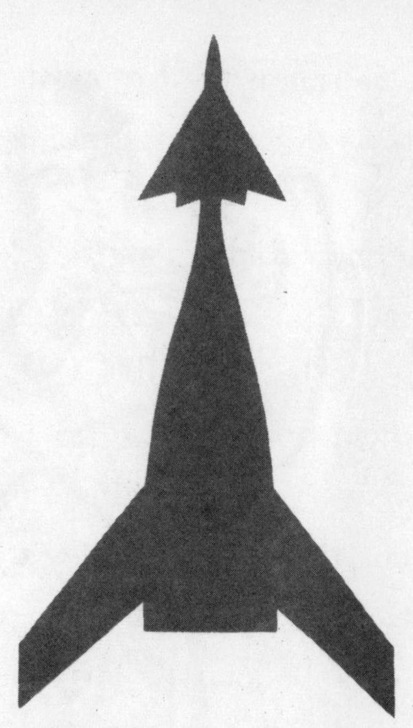

# 4

# MAKING A ROCKET GO FARTHER

Launching a big rocket is a wonderful thing to see.

Suppose you were watching a rocket in Florida. A tall crane lifts the rocket to the launching stand. The rocket stands as high as a seven-story building. There are scientific instruments in its nose.

About an hour before firing time, the fuel tanks

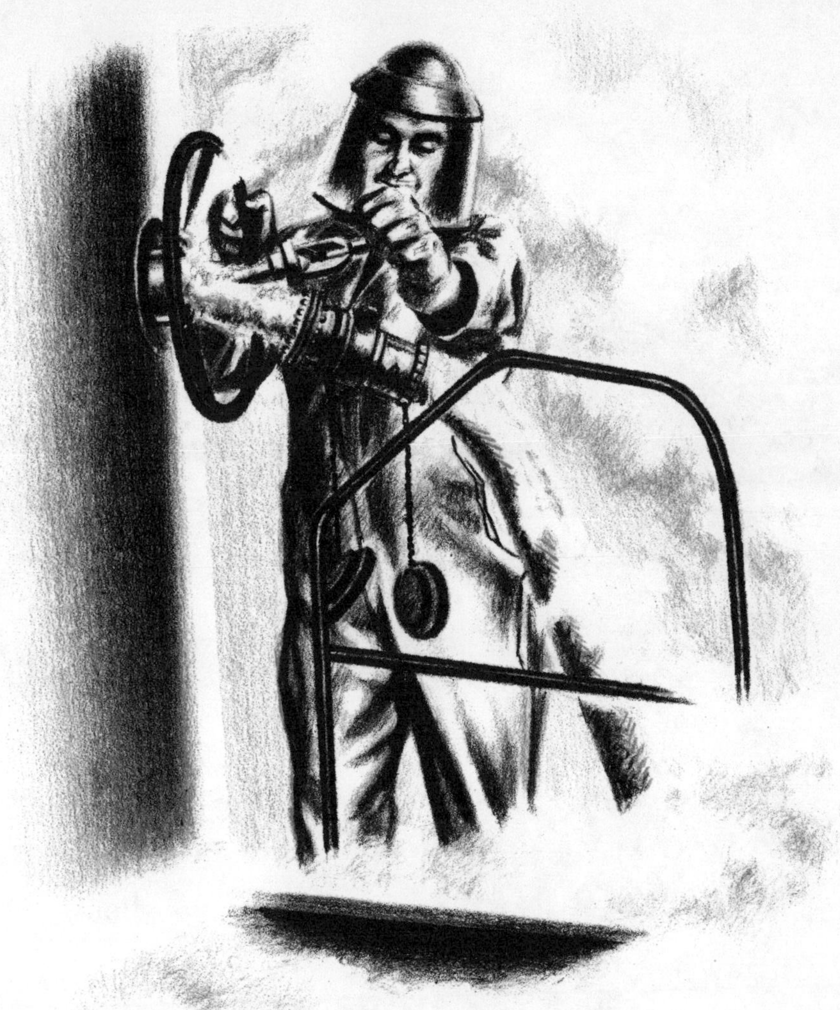

*Filling the fuel tanks is dangerous work.*

are filled. There is always danger of an explosion. The workmen wear special clothes to protect them from fire. They have hoods with plastic windows.

When the fuel tanks are full, the big crane moves

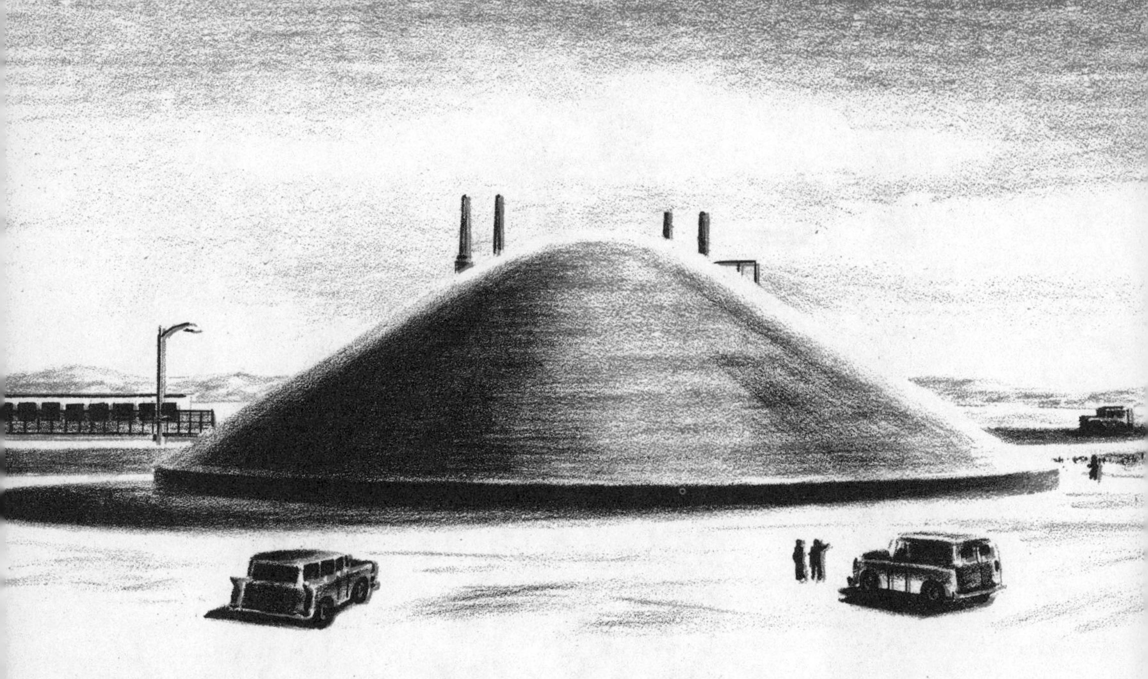

*Scientists and engineers work in the blockhouse.*

away on steel rails. The rocket stands alone. Wires go from the rocket to a concrete blockhouse hundreds of feet away. The outside of the blockhouse is many feet thick.

This blockhouse protects the scientists and engineers who fire the rocket. They will be safe inside if the rocket explodes or falls back. Everybody else must keep two miles away.

It is 10 minutes before firing time. In the blockhouse, the timekeeper begins to call off each min-

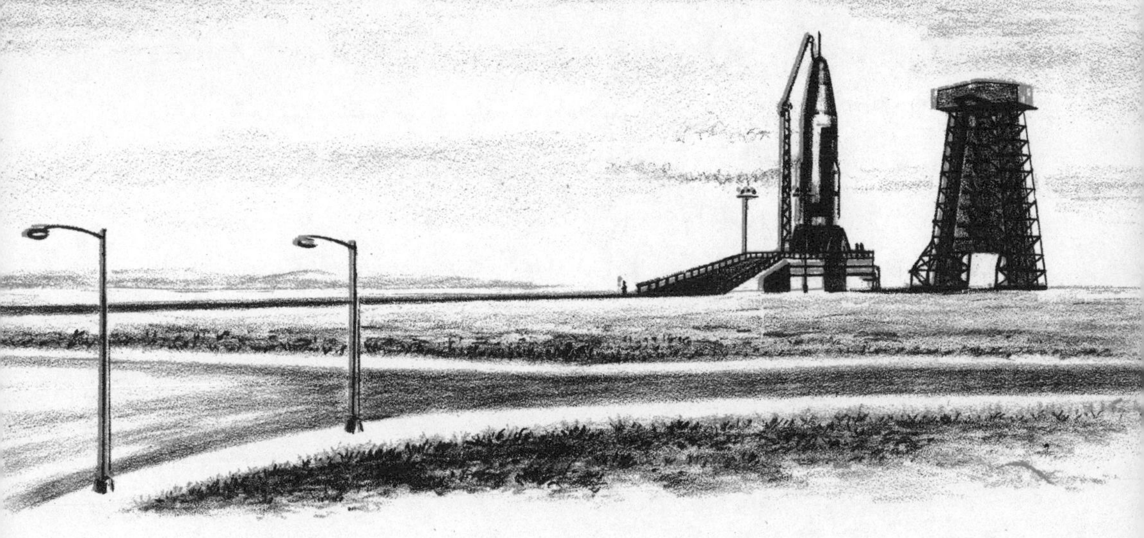

*The crane moves back from the rocket.*

ute. Scientists push different buttons to get the rocket ready for blasting off.

Meters show whether the rocket's delicate machinery is working as it should. The wires from the meters to the rocket will be cut off automatically when the rocket is fired.

The scientist in charge watches two rows of red and green lights. One by one the red lights change to green. This shows that all is working well inside the rocket.

The last light turns to green. This is the signal to the firing officer. He pushes a button that sends fuel into the rocket motor. Fire flashes from the bottom of the rocket with a tremendous roar.

In about two seconds, the rocket motor is burning with full power. Then the rocket rises from the launching stand. It shoots into the sky, leaving a stream of fire and smoke.

A rocket burns a huge amount of fuel in just a few seconds. It has to push through the thick blanket of air around the earth. And it must go very fast to overcome the pull of the earth's gravity.

Engineers have found a good way to get rockets into outer space. They build the rocket in parts called stages. A four-stage rocket has four different motors, one on top of the other.

The Juno II is a famous four-stage rocket. The motor of the first stage is at the tail end. It carries the rocket about 60 miles high in about 3 minutes. All the fuel is burned. A radio signal from the ground cuts off the first stage from the rest of the rocket. It falls back into the ocean. The other three stages keep coasting on up.

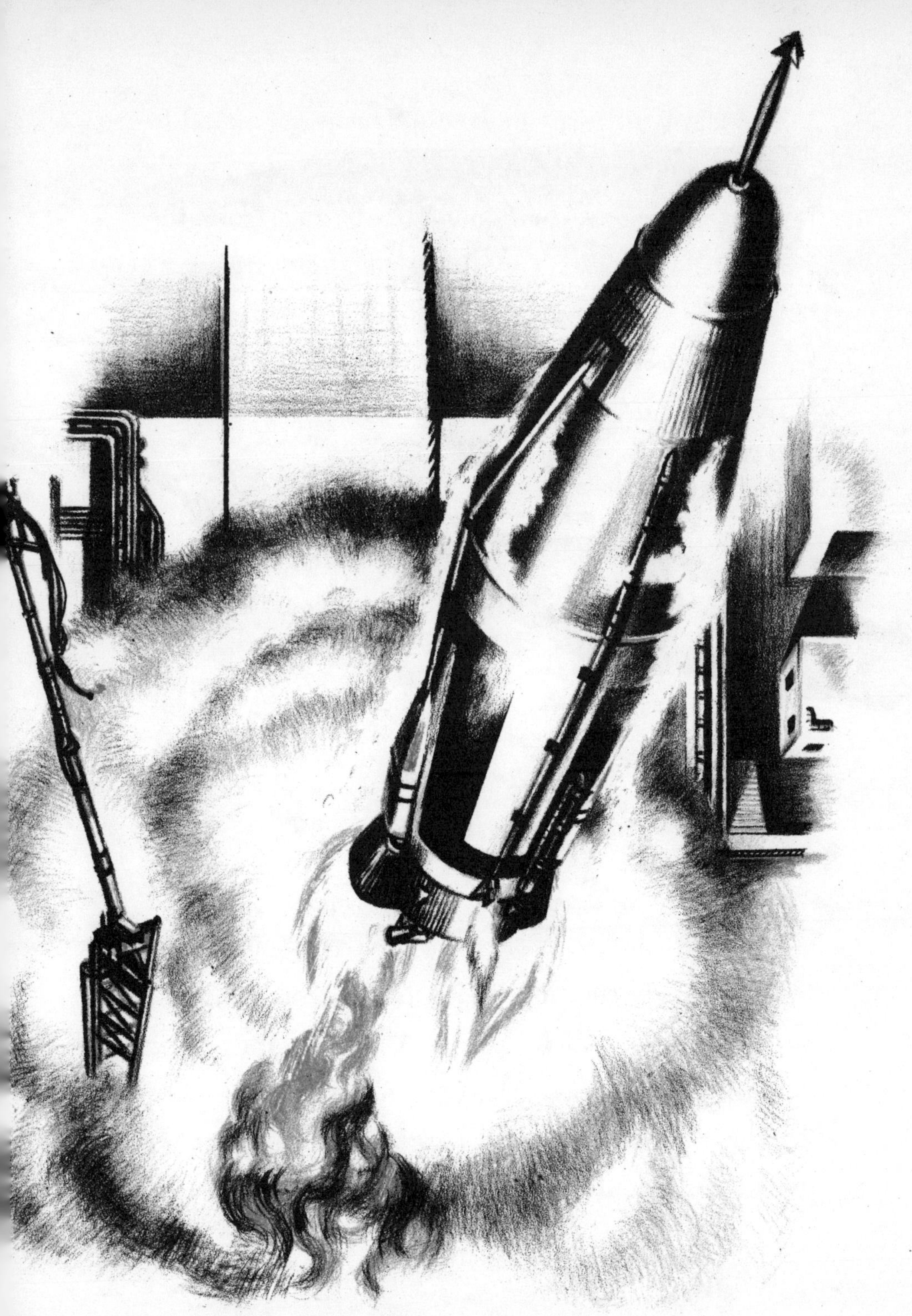

*In a few seconds the rocket begins to rise.*

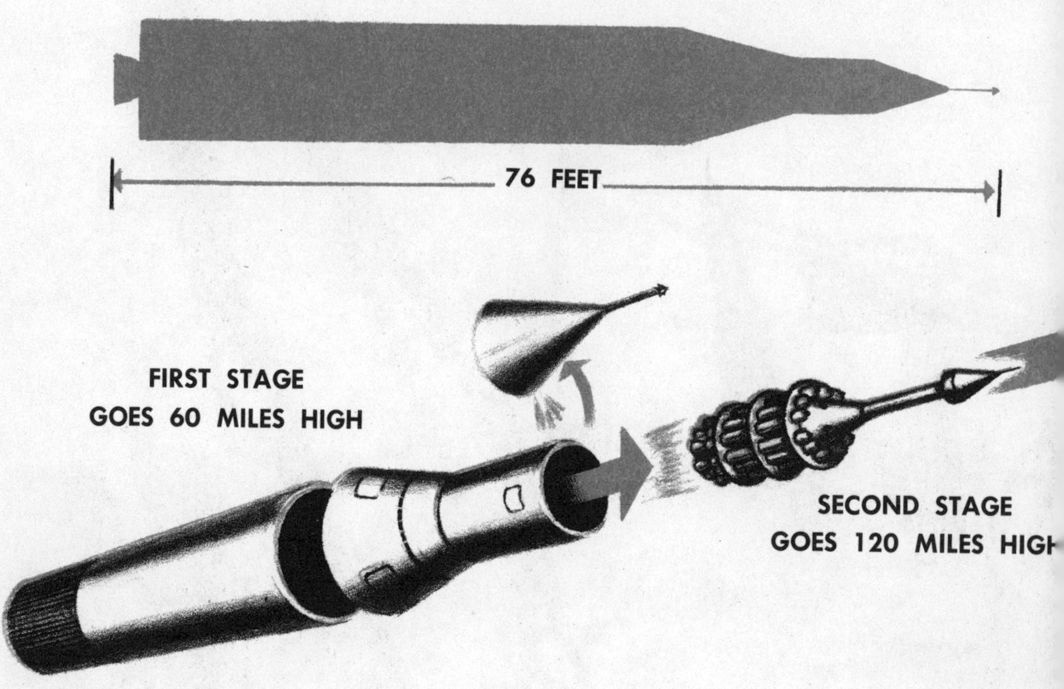


*The Juno II rocket has four stages.*

Next the motor of the second stage begins to fire. The fuel is burned up in 9 seconds. But the rocket is now going much faster. Another radio signal cuts this motor loose. The second stage falls away.

The third and fourth stages fire for only 9 seconds, too. But they give two more big pushes. Now

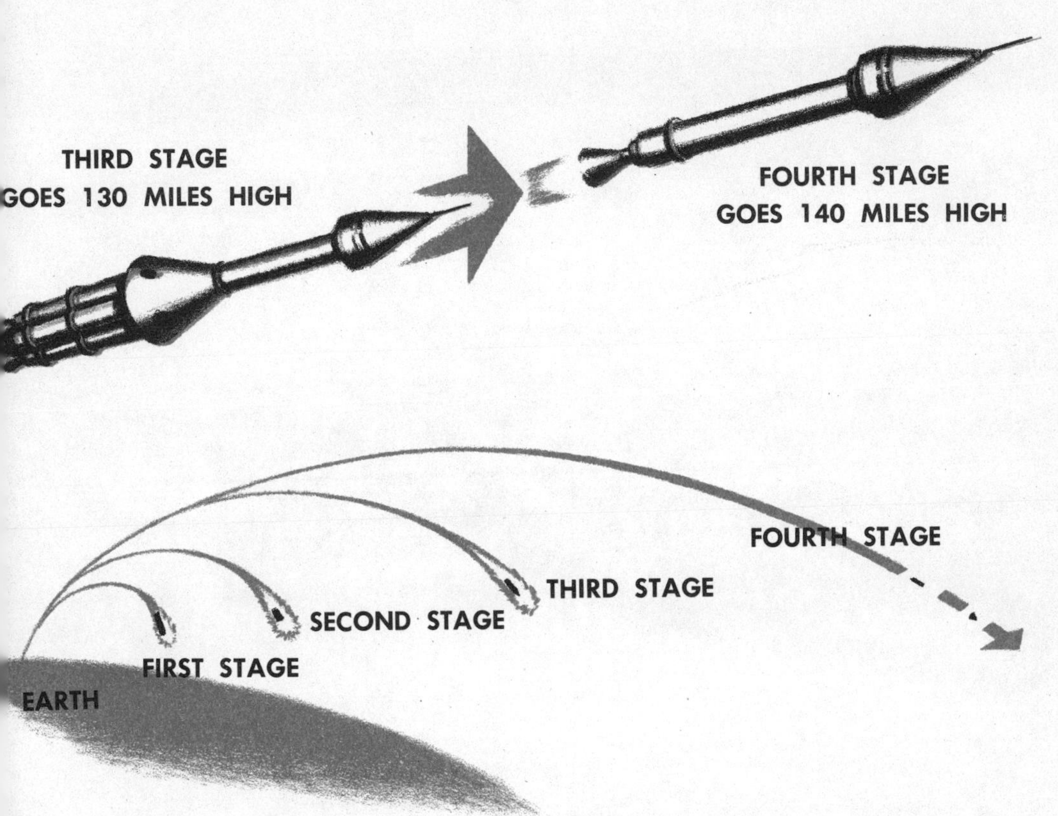


*The first three stages drop off quickly.*

the fourth stage is going fast enough to escape from the earth's gravity.

How fast is that? The speed is almost 25,000 miles an hour. If you went from New York to California at that speed, your trip would take only 7 minutes.

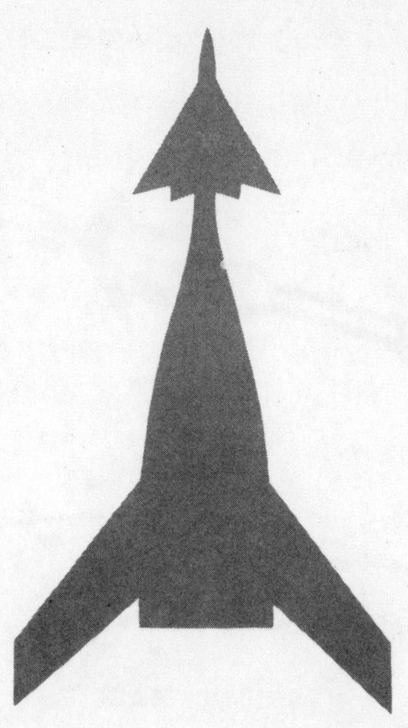

# 5

# WHAT A SATELLITE IS

The satellite we know best is the moon. It follows the earth as we travel around the sun. The moon is always circling the earth. It goes all the way around us once every 27 days.

The path of a satellite is called its orbit. Why does a satellite like the moon keep circling the earth?

Why doesn't the moon disappear into outer space?

The earth pulls things to itself. This pull is gravity. The earth holds the moon in an orbit around it.

The earth will also keep a small man-made satellite circling around it. A rocket shoots the satellite into outer space. A large satellite needs a huge rocket. The rocket must be about 1,000 times heavier than the satellite.

Even a small satellite can carry scientific instruments and a radio. It can send reports on temperatures and cosmic rays.

The first man-made satellite was launched Octo-

*The moon circles the earth. Both circle the sun.*

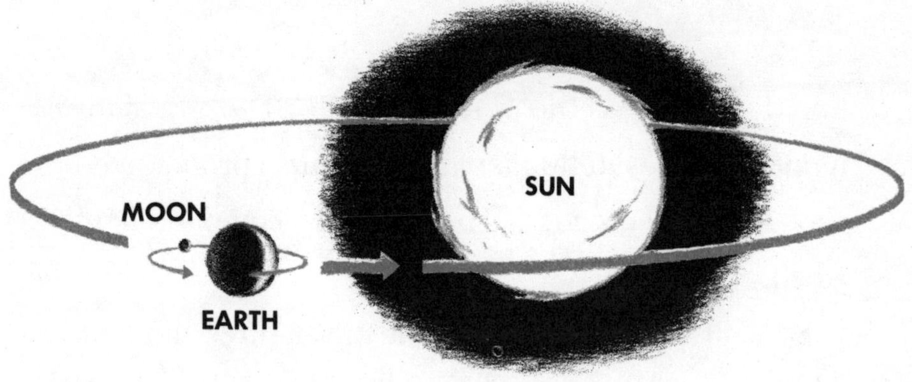

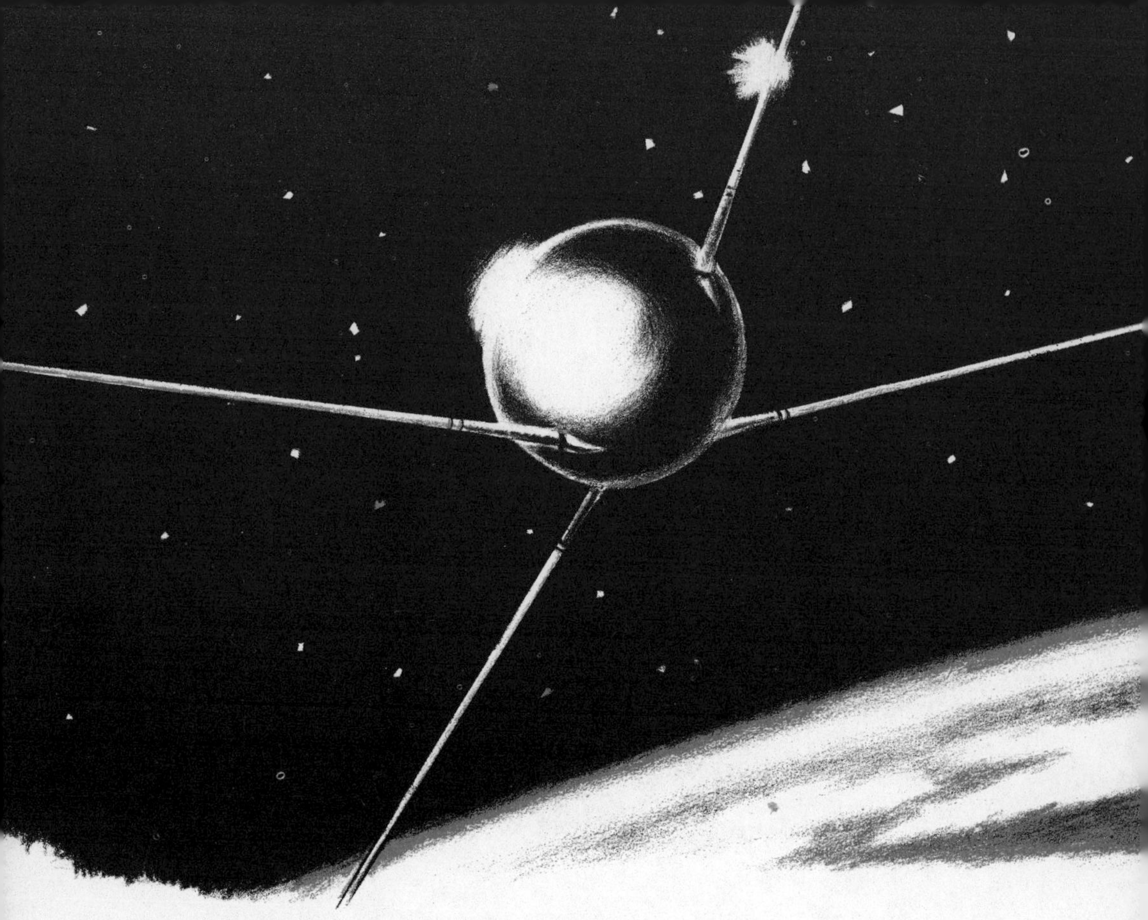

*Sputnik No. 1 was the first man-made satellite.*

ber 4, 1957, by the Soviet Union. The Russians named their satellite *sputnik zemli* (pronounced SPOOT-nick zem-LEE). That means "companion of earth."

Sputnik No. 1 circled the earth for three months. All this time it was sinking closer to the earth. It

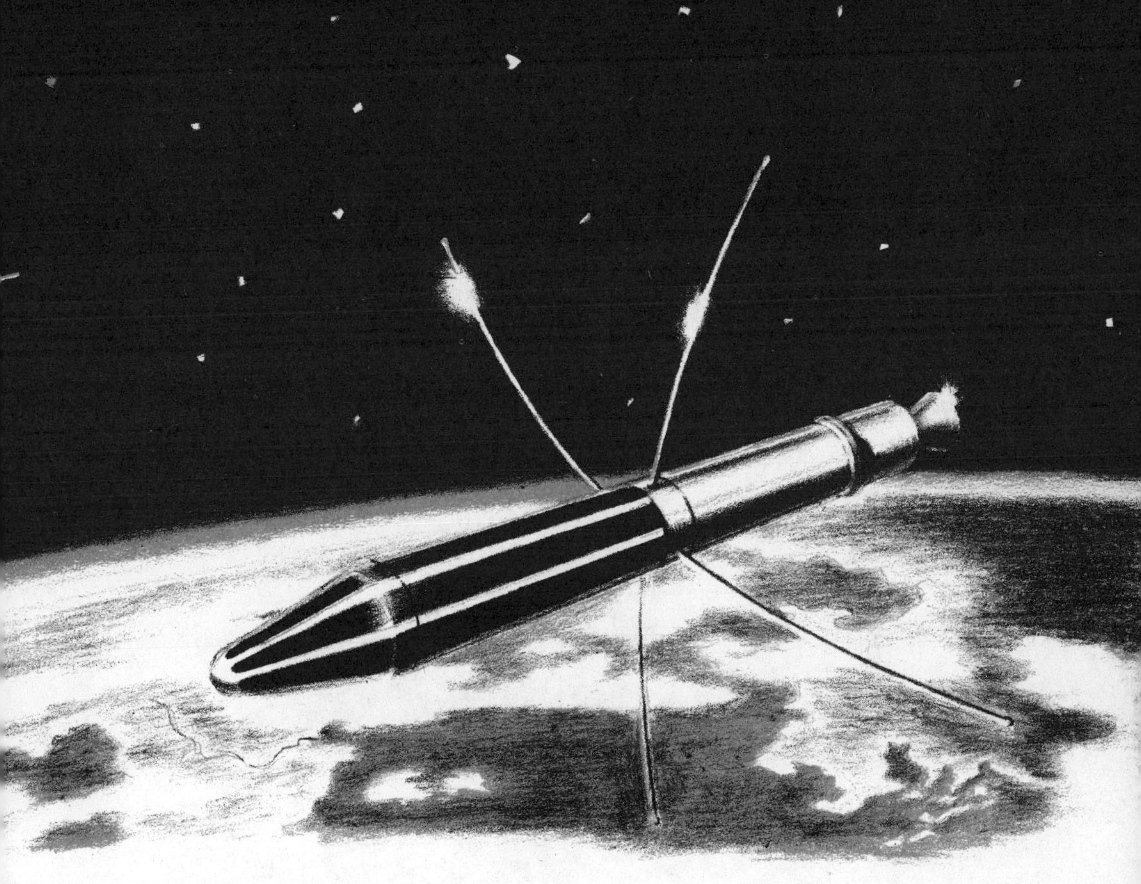

*The first American satellite was Explorer I.*

finally burned up when it came down into thick air a few miles above us.

Why did it catch fire? Because of friction. Friction means rubbing together. Two pieces of wood will get very hot if you rub them together rapidly. They will even begin to burn.

Almost anything will catch fire if it goes through ordinary air at terrific speed.

The Russians shot a second Sputnik into space on November 3, 1957. This was the first satellite to carry a live animal. The famous passenger was a dog

*A receiving station picks up signals from satellites.*

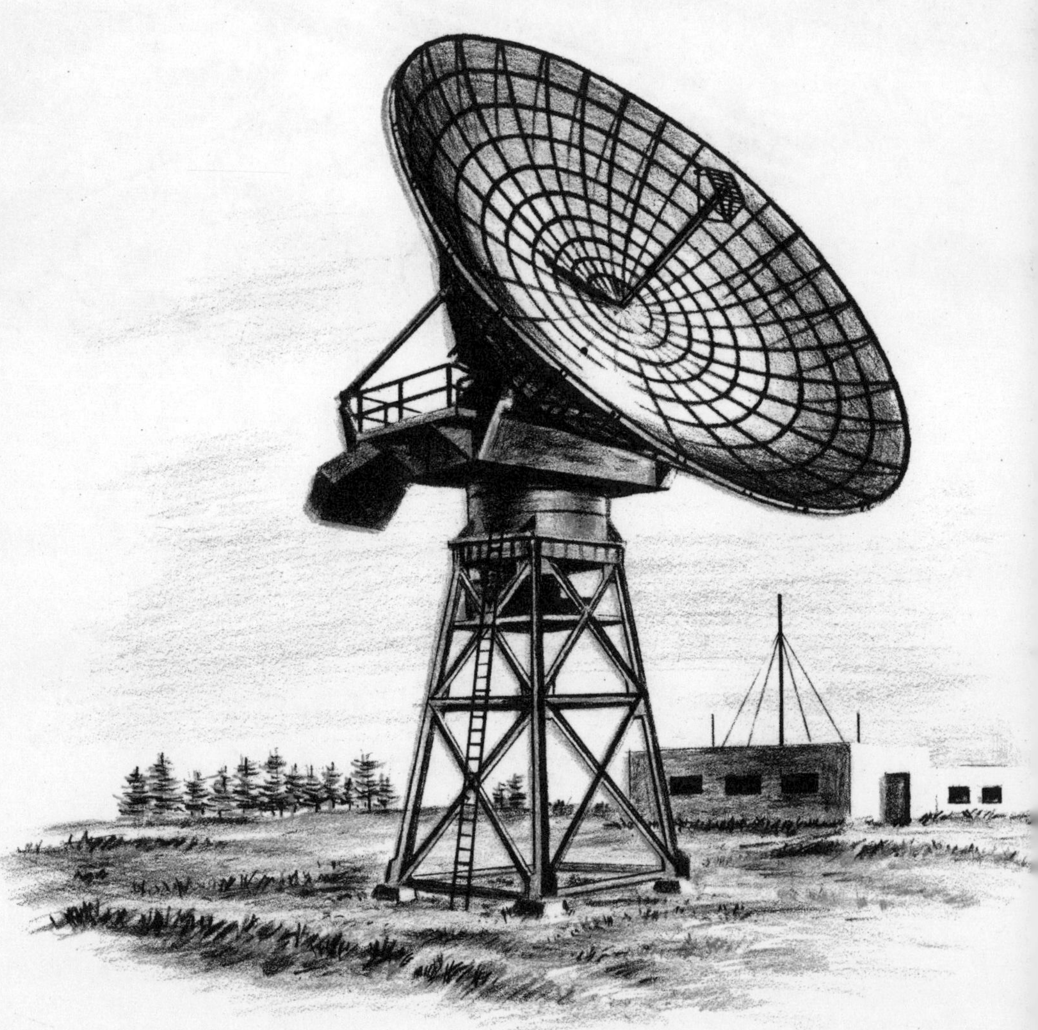

named Laika. The dog lived for three or four days. It was put to death painlessly.

Why was a dog sent into outer space? Because men want to go there, too. First we must find out whether an animal can stay alive in space.

The first American satellite was called Explorer I. It was shot into space on January 31, 1958. A four-stage rocket was used. The launching was from the rocket base at Cape Canaveral, Florida. In less than 7 minutes, the satellite was in orbit far above the earth.

Explorer I weighed 31 pounds. The space inside a small satellite must be used very carefully. All of the instruments must be tiny. The radio is very small. But it can send a signal 4,000 miles.

Receiving stations on the earth pick up the radio signals. Each *beep-beep* signal tells something. Signals change to report different facts from outer space.

A little satellite travels fast. It can circle the earth in less than two hours.

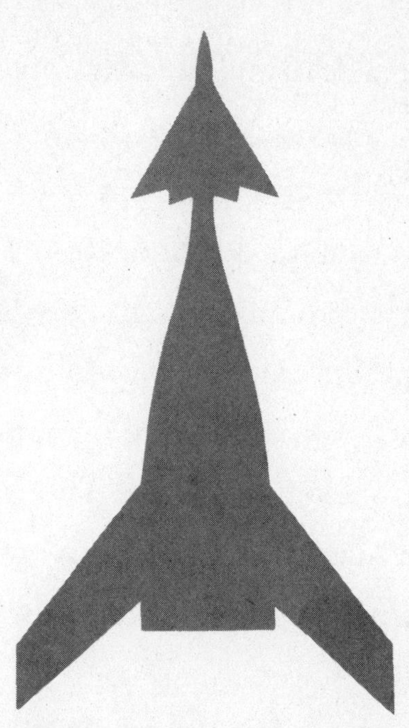

# 6

# PUTTING A MAN INTO SPACE

We now have man-made satellites going around the earth and sun. Very soon a satellite may be going around the moon.

The next big job is to send a man into space. He will travel inside a satellite. His satellite will be shot into space by a giant rocket.

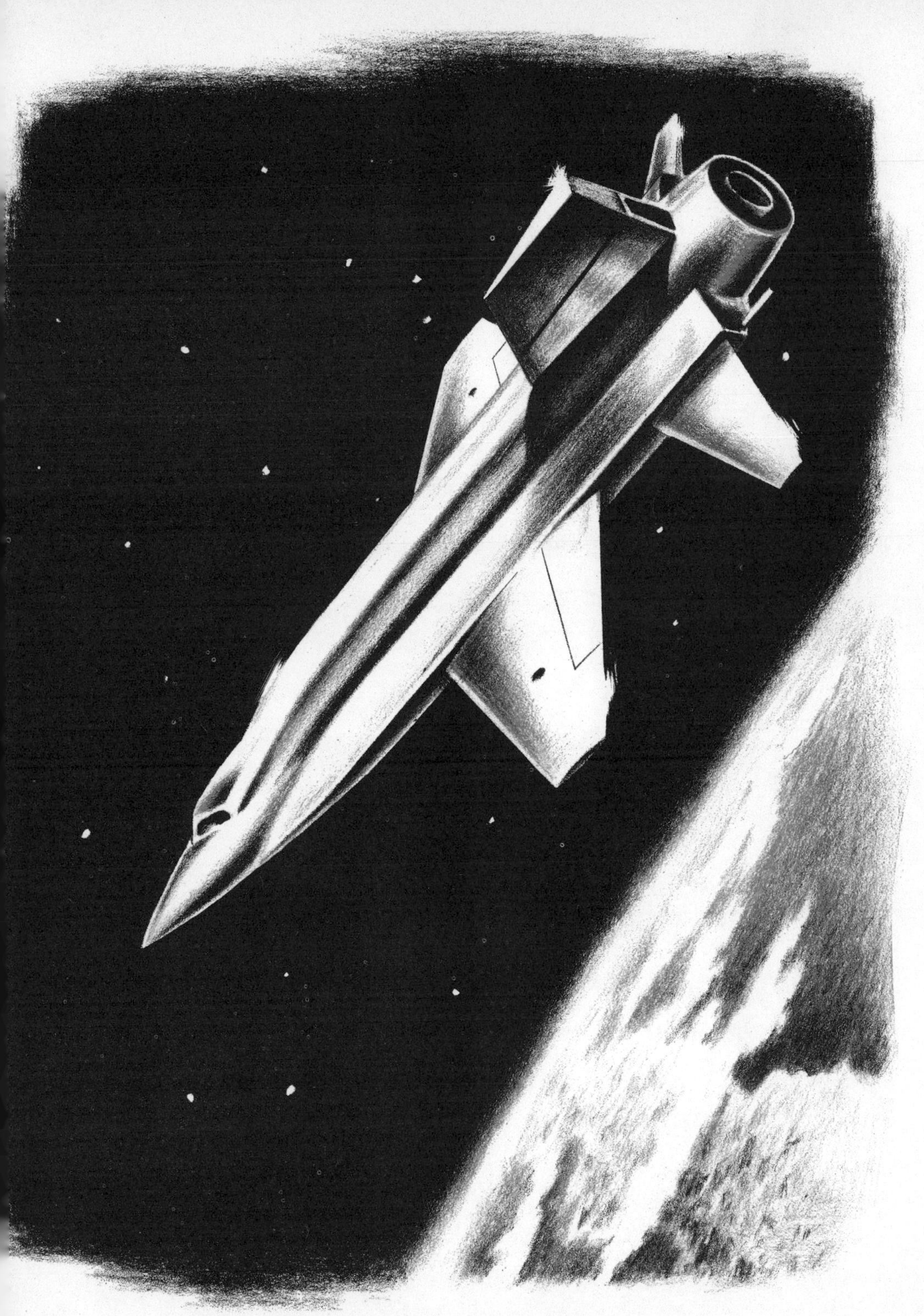

*The X-15 takes off from a high-flying plane.*

It will be fairly easy to build this giant rocket. The hard problem is building a satellite or space ship for the passenger.

We must build a space ship that can come back safely. It must not burn up when it strikes the earth's air blanket. It must go slowly enough to keep from catching fire.

Scientists are drawing plans for a space ship that can return to earth. Perhaps it will have wings like a high-speed airplane. Then it can glide through the air gradually.

The space ship may use small rockets for brakes. The rockets would fire toward the front, not the back. They would slow down the ship as it neared the earth.

Another problem is the take-off. What will happen to the man inside when a rocket leaves the ground? You know how it feels when an automobile starts with a jerk. You are thrown back against the seat.

A rocket starts ever so much faster. Could the pilot breathe? Suppose he fainted? Then what?

Scientists are studying these questions. They are

making many tests. They have a special machine that spins a man around very fast at the end of a long steel beam. The man on the beam feels the way a rocket passenger would feel.

In the test a man can breathe easily. He does not faint if he is lying down.

Rocket passengers will not sit up during take-offs. They will lie down for a few minutes. Each person's body will seem very heavy.

*A one-man space ship may look like this.*

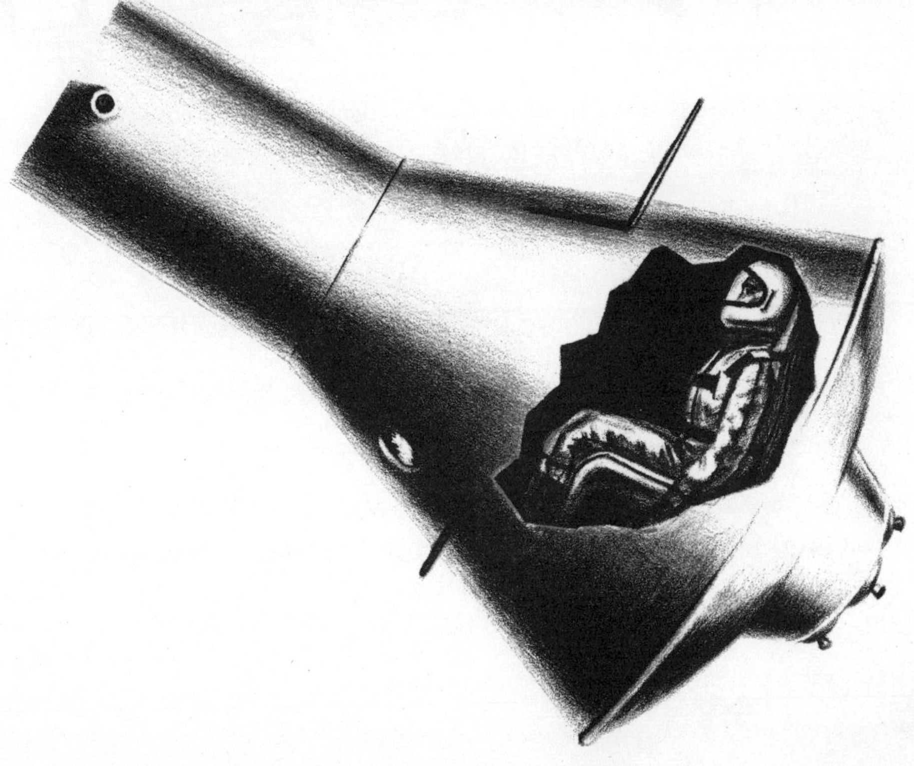

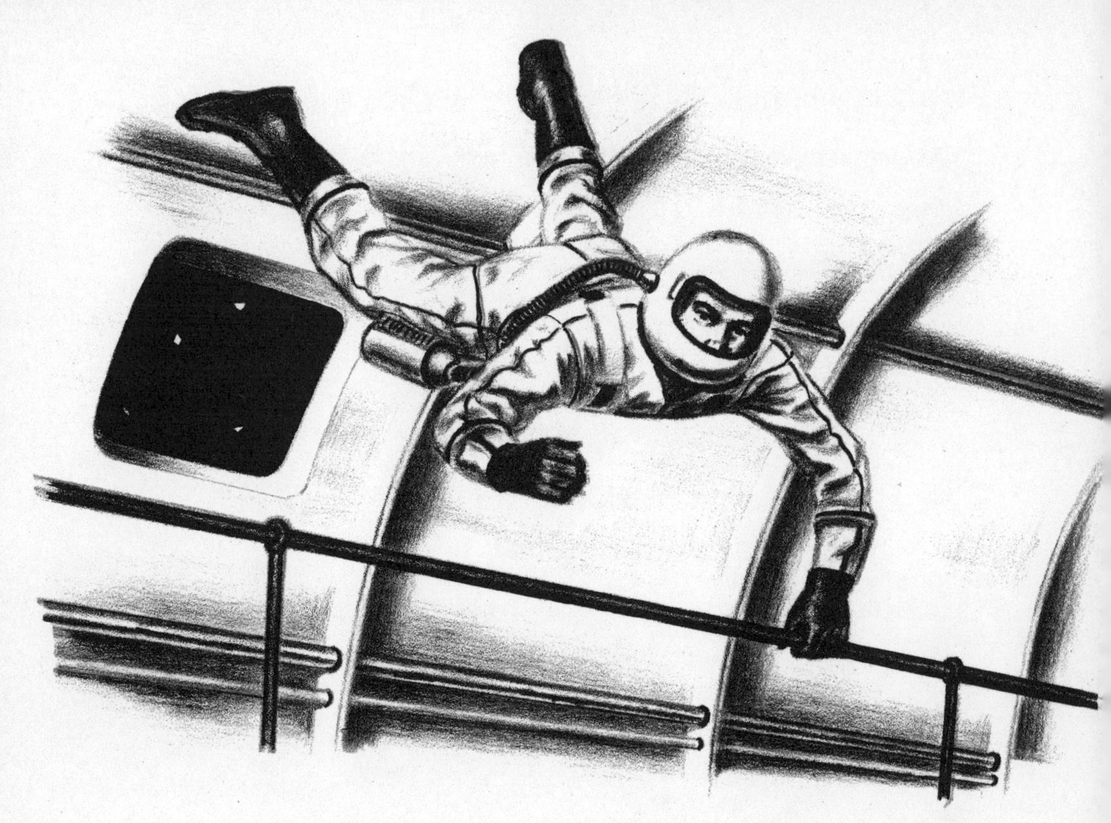

*Without gravity, a man would float like a leaf.*

Then the rocket motors will be shut off, and the rocket will coast in space. What a different feeling then! The passengers won't have any weight at all. Nothing will have any weight.

Suppose you were a passenger and held a coin in your fist. If you opened your fingers, the coin would float in air. It would not fall to the floor.

You would have a hard time trying to eat or drink. Food wouldn't stay on your fork. If you picked up a glass of water, you couldn't drink it. The water wouldn't run into your mouth. It would form a ball and go somewhere else.

These things happen when you get beyond the pull of gravity. Gravity makes rivers run downhill. It makes water run down your throat.

Gravity gets weaker as you get farther from the earth. In outer space, you can't feel any pull from the earth.

Probably the first space traveler will make only a short trip. He may come back in a few hours. But in that time he will circle the earth several times.

He will follow an orbit as the small satellites are doing now. He will bring back thousands of photographs of the earth and moon. His instruments will have new facts for scientists to study.

Everything he learns will help in planning longer flights into space.

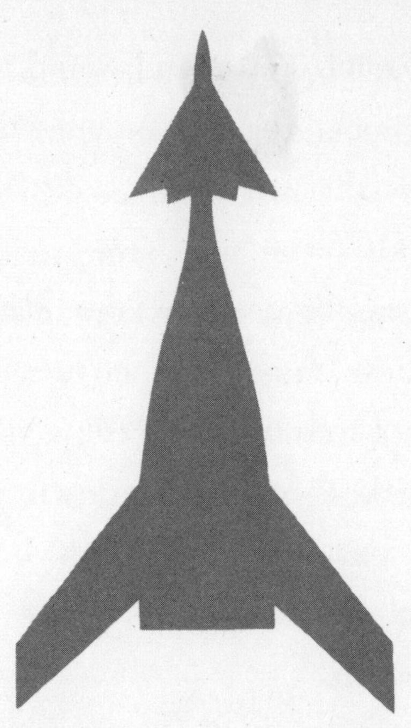

# 7

# BUILDING A SPACE STATION

The first man in space will be about 500 to 1,000 miles up. He will circle the earth at about 18,000 miles an hour.

Later a space station will be built that far up. It will go around the earth like a satellite.

There are many plans for the first space station. Dr. Wernher von Braun has planned a station like a big wheel. The wheel would be almost as wide as a city block. The entrance would be at the hub. People would walk through large, hollow spokes to the rim.

Inside the rim would be machine shops and laboratories. There would be rooms where engineers and scientists would live. There would be storage rooms for food, water, and even air.

The space station would be built on the ground. After being tested, it would be taken apart. The steel girders and walls would be carried into space by giant rockets.

*This space station could be as wide as a city block.*

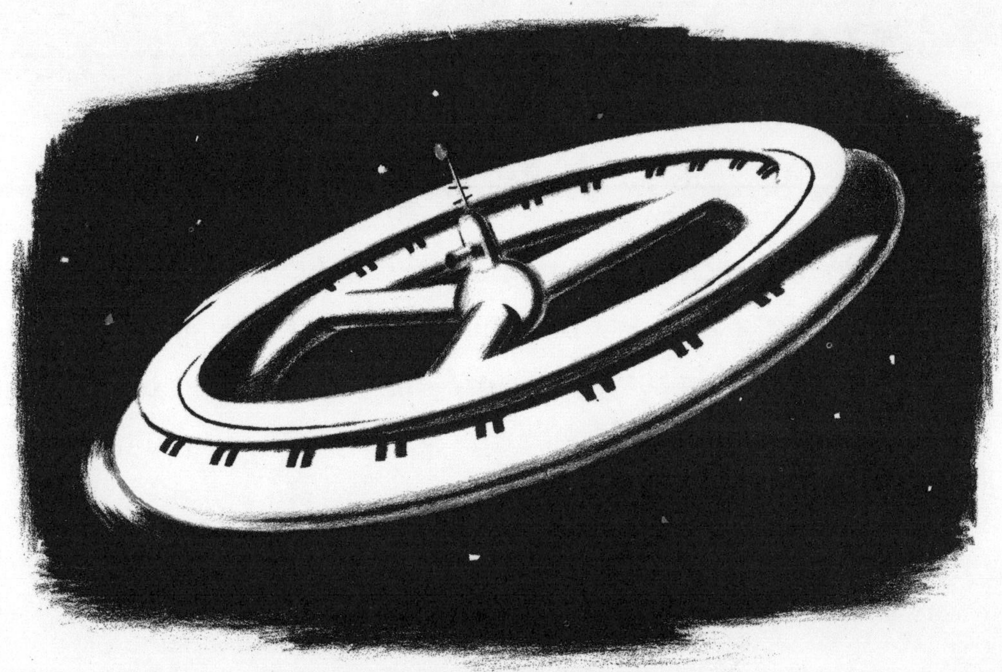

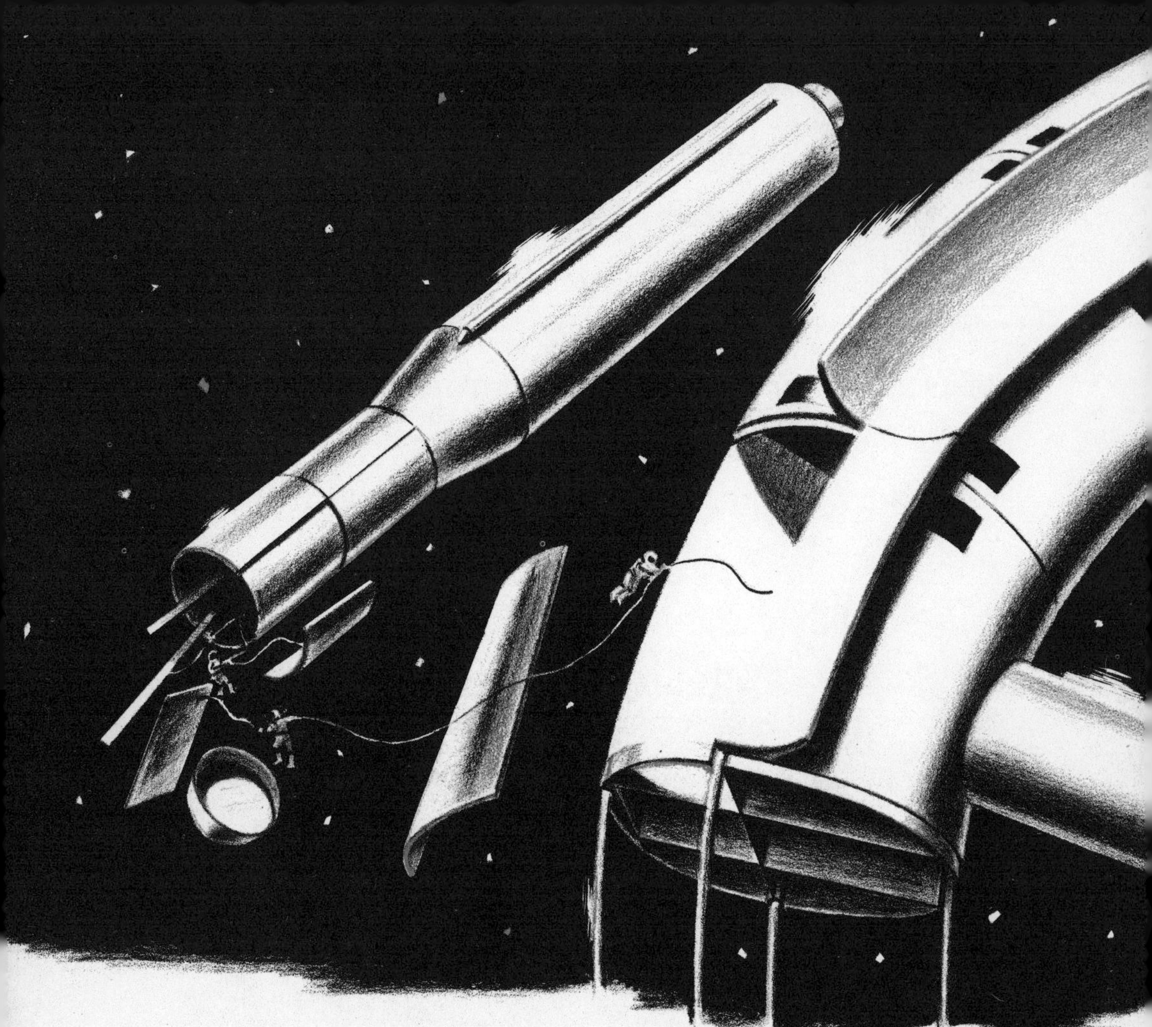

*Materials for the station will float in space.*

When each rocket reached the right height, the building materials would be pushed out into space. They wouldn't fall because they would be beyond the pull of the earth's gravity. They would behave like satellites.

They would circle the earth at 18,000 miles an hour. They would travel as fast as the rocket.

Men in space suits would step out of the rocket. They wouldn't fall, either. But they would have ropes fastened to them so they couldn't drift away. The building materials would have to be tied on, too.

Engineers and mechanics would put the space station together. One man could handle the biggest girder because it would be weightless.

There will never be rain or snow or clouds at the space station. Crew members will see where storms are beginning on earth. They will watch the oceans and the frozen wastes around the North and South Poles. Every day they will send radio reports to weathermen on earth.

The space station will be a wonderful place to study the sun, moon, and stars. The sky will be black, not blue. The sun and millions of other stars will shine brilliantly. Nothing will spoil the view.

A space ship to the moon might take off from

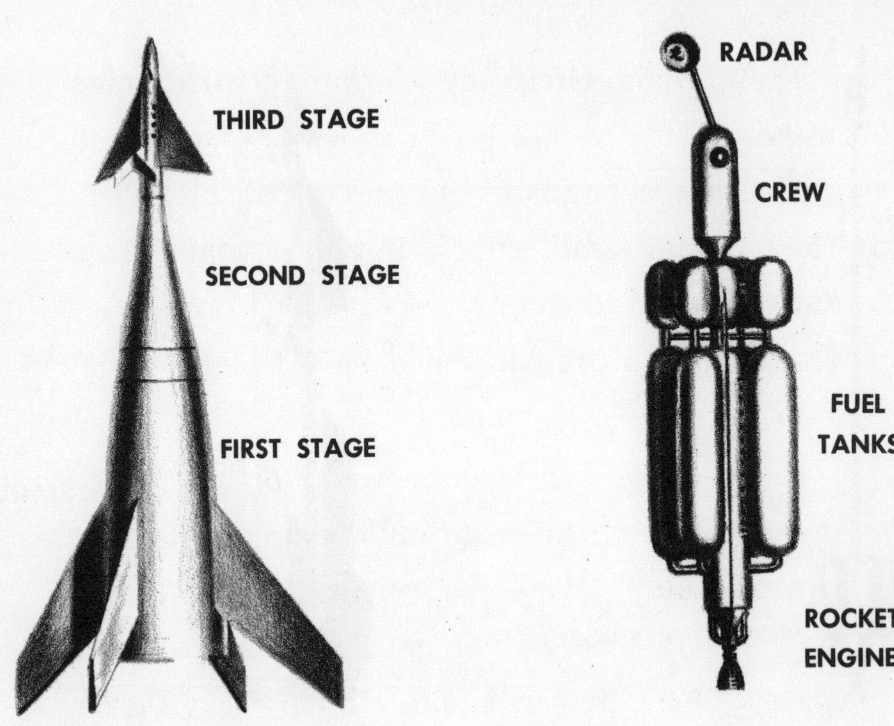


*Plans are being drawn for different space ships.*

the space station. In fact, it might be built at the station. This would be very different from a space ship that must come back to earth. It wouldn't need wings. It could be very light. It wouldn't have to carry a huge amount of fuel for its rockets.

This is because outer space has no air to slow down the space ship. Another reason is that the ship will get a flying start. The space station will

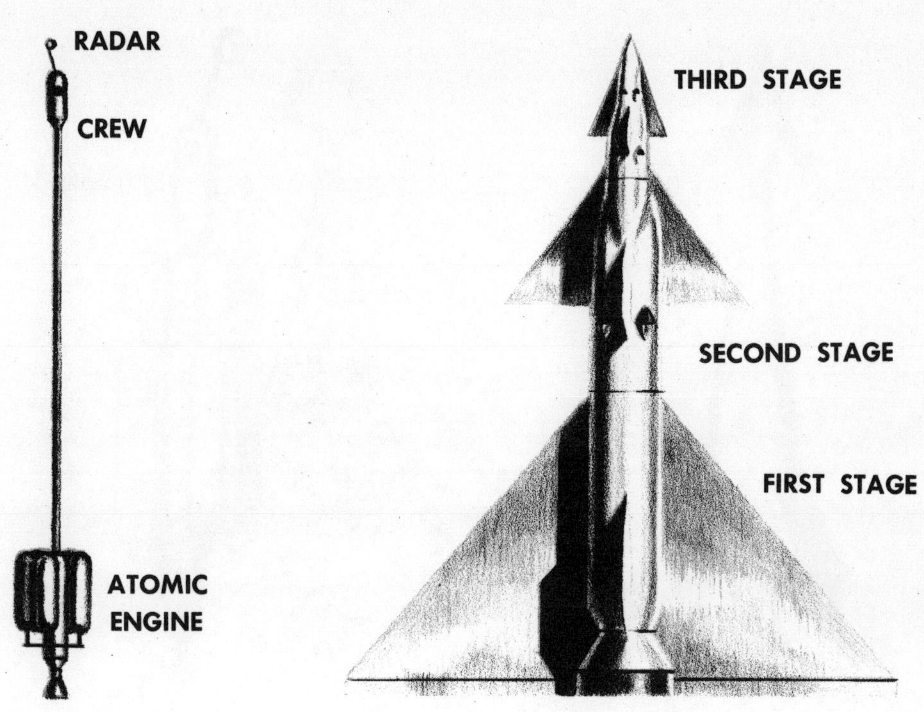


*These four drawings show how different they are.*

always travel at about 18,000 miles an hour. So the space ship will be going that fast *before* it takes off. It will need to go some 23,000 miles an hour to reach the moon. Getting the extra speed won't take much fuel.

The space ship might be an open steel framework with a cabin. It might be a large ball with spidery legs. Or it might be shaped like a rocket.

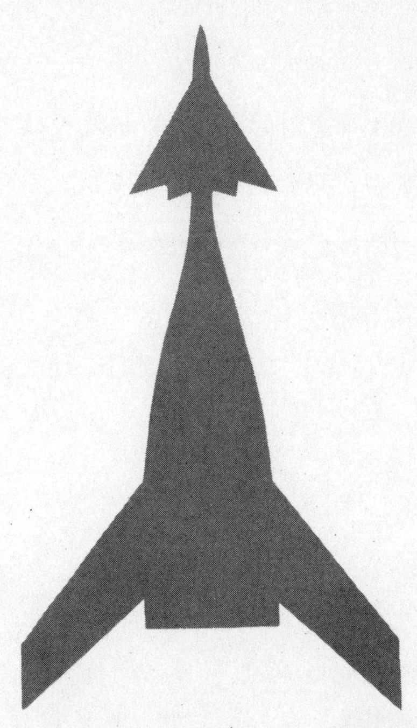

# 8

# DANGERS IN SPACE

Living in a space station and flying by space ship will have many dangers.

One of the dangers is a flying piece of rock or metal, usually no bigger than a pebble. It is called a meteor.

A meteor whizzes through space at 40 miles a

second. That is faster than a rifle bullet. When the meteor strikes the air blanket around the earth, it burns up from friction. Then you see the flash of fire. It is called a "shooting star."

There is a steady rain of meteors in outer space. Most of them are smaller than a grain of sand. They wouldn't even dent the stainless-steel wall of the space station. But many thousands could gradually wear the wall away.

Probably the space station will have two walls. The outer wall will be a shield against meteors. When it wears thin, it will be replaced.

You may wonder where meteors come from. They

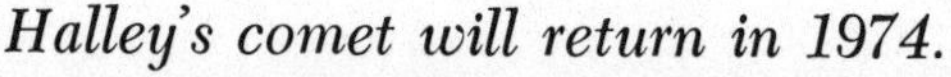

*Halley's comet will return in 1974.*

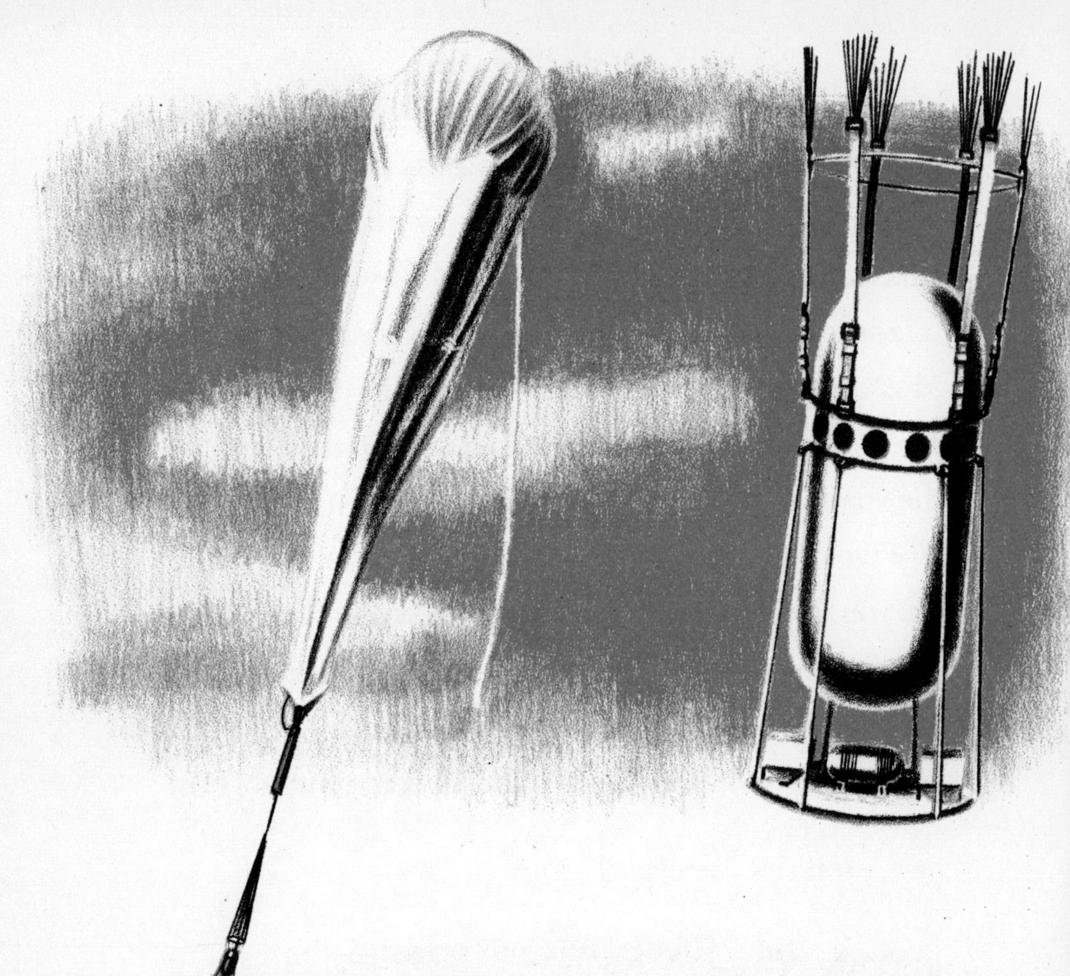

*Skyhook balloons can go 20 miles high.*

are the tiny pieces of comets that have broken up. A comet looks like a star with a tail. It circles the sun.

In 1910 Halley's comet came very close to the earth. Its long, gassy tail actually swept across the earth—without hurting anyone. This same comet will return in 1974. Don't forget.

Another danger in outer space is cosmic rays. Nobody knows yet exactly where they come from. These rays are deadly. They are something like X-rays. On earth we are protected from cosmic rays by our blanket of air. What about man in space? Can he be protected?

The U.S. Air Force made an experiment to find out. It sent a big Skyhook balloon, made of thin plastic, 20 miles into the sky. At that height there is practically no air.

The balloon carried a passenger in a gondola. He was Major David C. Simons, a doctor. Major Simons stayed up for 32 hours. He came back in good health. The cosmic rays hadn't hurt him. Scientists believe that men can be protected anywhere in space.

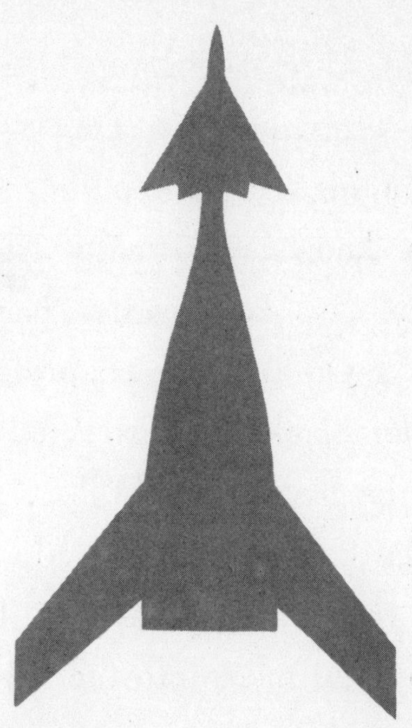

# 9

# GETTING TO THE MOON

A trip to the moon will be a great adventure in the exploration of space.

Some scientists think we'll get to the moon in a few years. Others say it will take longer. But all agree it will be done.

The trip may be made in two stages. The first

stage would be from earth to a space station. The second stage would be from the space station to the moon.

It would cost a lot of money to buy a ticket to the moon. If you had a ticket, you would go to the rocket launching field. There you would take an elevator to the cabin of a huge rocket.

Before the rocket motors start, your seat will be tilted back to make a bed. When you are lying down, you won't feel the rocket's speed so much.

In a few minutes you will be 500 miles up. Your

*A space traveler will lie down for the take-off.*

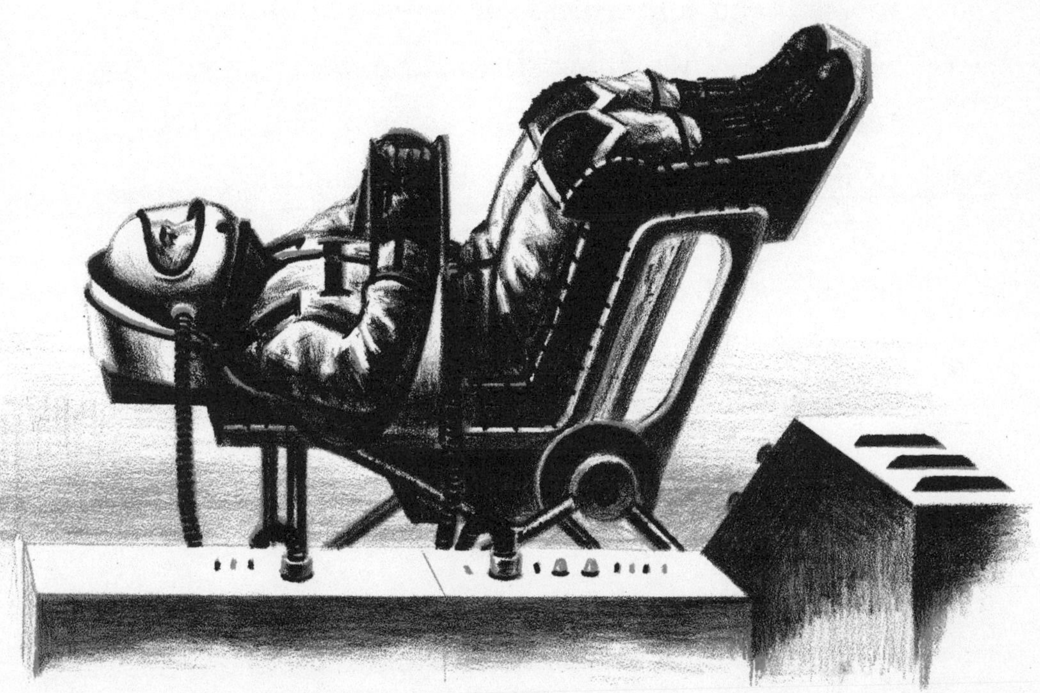

rocket may circle the earth a few times. Then you will come to the space station. You will spend an hour or so at the space station. It will be exciting to look down at the earth through telescopes.

A space ship smaller than the big rocket from earth will be waiting for passengers. It will take you on the long journey to the moon.

The rocket motors of your ship will fire for just a few minutes to build up speed. Then for three days you will coast through space. In these three days you will travel 240,000 miles.

Ahead of you the moon will seem to grow larger and larger. You will see several dark areas on the moon. Long ago astronomers thought these were oceans. Now we know there is no water or air on the moon. The dark areas are actually long stretches of flat land surrounded by high mountains.

Perhaps your pilot won't head straight for a landing. Instead he will fire his rockets for a few moments. This will steer the ship into position to circle the moon.

About 200 miles from the moon, you will get a

thrilling view. The moon's craters will be in plain sight. Perhaps you have seen photographs of them. The pictures are made with powerful telescopes.

Some of the moon's craters are so small you can barely see them from the space ship. The biggest are more than 100 miles across. Every now and then you will see a mountain in the middle of a crater.

You will notice light-colored streaks running out many miles from some craters. They look like rays —and that is what astronomers call them. They will remind you of highways going out from a city. But

*Some of the moon's craters are 100 miles across.*

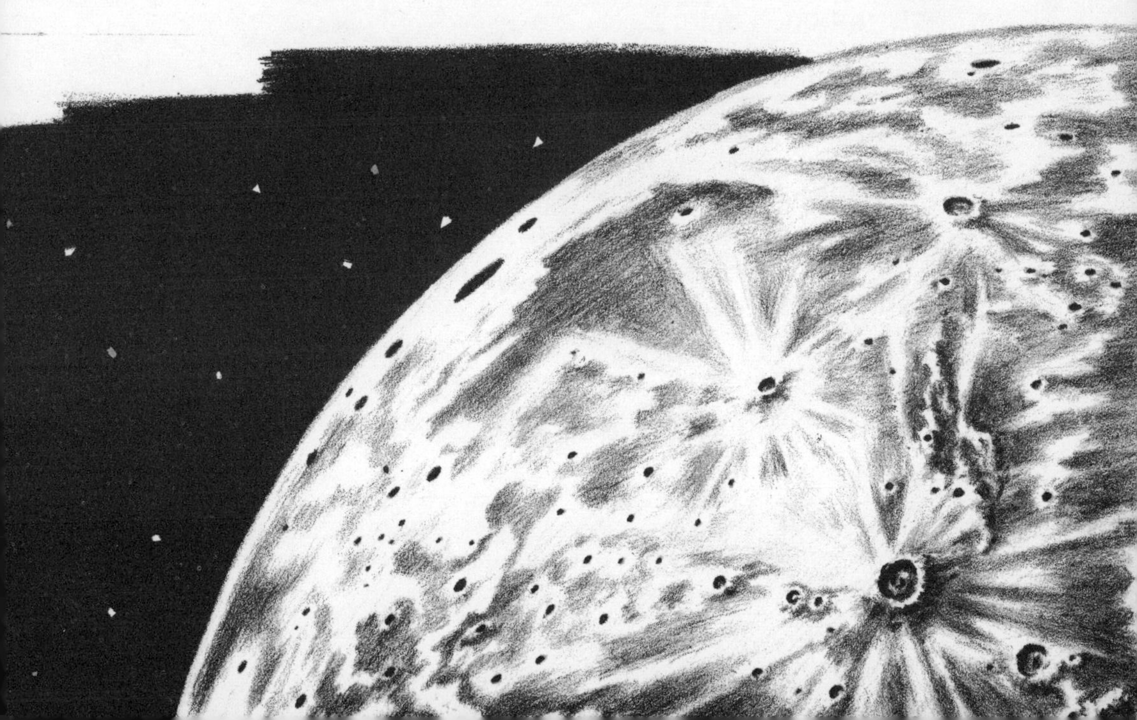

the moon has no cities and no highways. No one knows what caused these rays.

Soon you will get a view that we cannot get from the earth. You will see the other side of the moon. The moon always turns the same face toward the earth. We don't know what the other side looks like. Probably it has great plains, tall mountains, and many craters, too. We can be sure there are no green fields with cows and sheep.

The moon is not the place for a pleasant vacation. Daylight on the moon lasts for two weeks. The sun

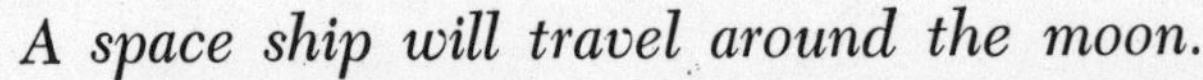

*A space ship will travel around the moon.*

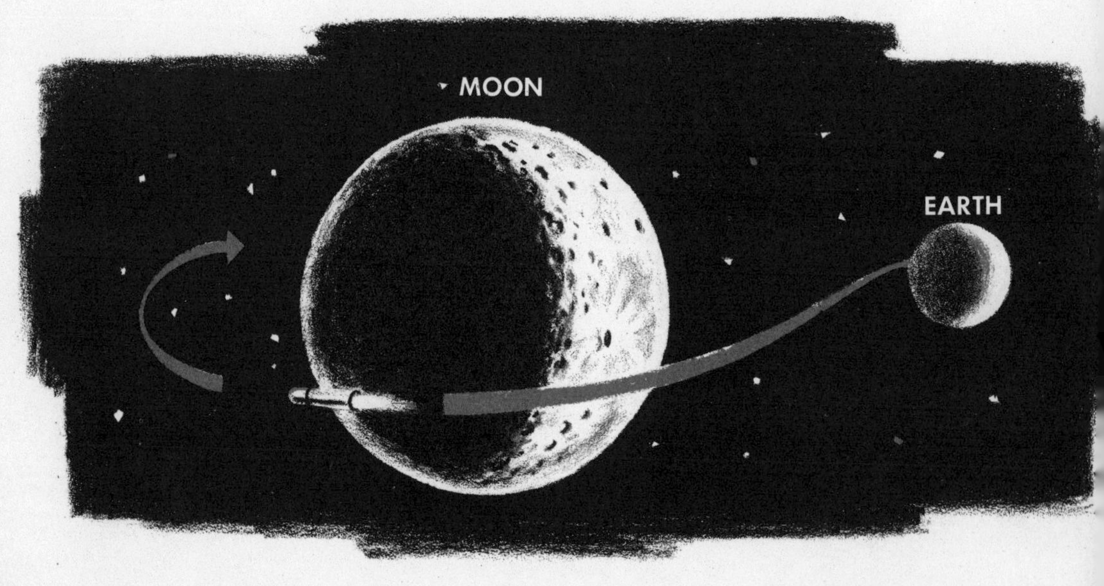

keeps heating the bare rocks and dusty ground until the moon gets as hot as boiling water.

Darkness on the moon also lasts two weeks. During the long night the place gets colder than you can imagine—more than 200 degrees below zero.

Your space ship will come down on one of the broad, flat plains. Before you step out of the ship, you will have to get into an air-conditioned space suit. You could not stand the heat without it. Your suit will have a small oxygen tank so that you can breathe. It will be a thick suit, almost like armor. That is to protect you from the tiny meteors that whiz through space.

How can you walk around in a suit weighing a lot more than you do? On the moon the suit won't seem heavy at all. That's because the moon is much smaller than the earth and has much less gravity.

The pull of gravity on the moon is only one-sixth of what you feel on earth. A space suit weighing 300 pounds on earth would weigh only 50 pounds on the moon.

Of course you would weigh less, too. You would

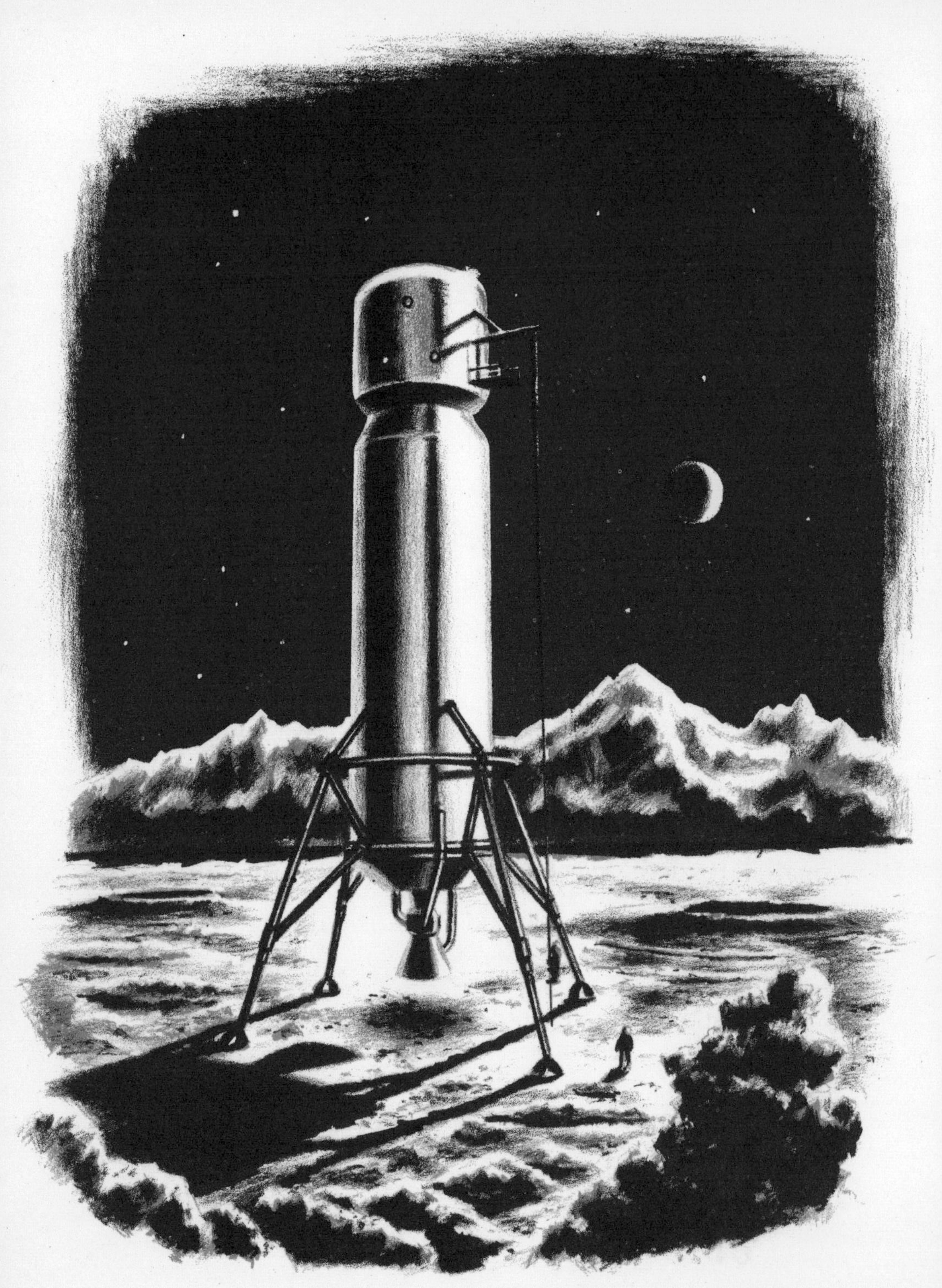

*Visitors to the moon will land on a broad plain.*

weigh so little you could jump over a two-story house—if you happened to find one. It would be wise not to try any big jumps. You might come down on a sharp rock that would tear a hole in your space suit. All the air would pass out. You would pass out, too.

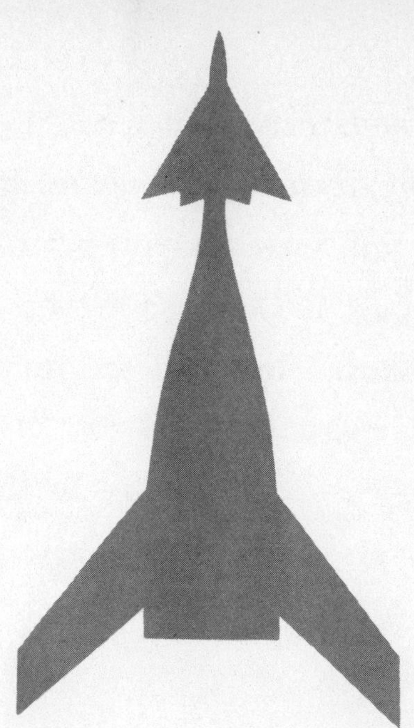

# 10
# LIVING ON THE MOON

Before many years pass, several hundred people may be living on the moon.

How can they live in a place that has no air or water? How will they keep from freezing during the long nights? How will they protect themselves from the sun's fierce heat?

Scientists have answers to these questions. They know that men can live underground. Most of their work will be done underground, too.

Rooms and workshops will be carved out of the solid rock. They will be air-conditioned and bright with electric lights. Below ground there will be no danger from the rain of meteors.

An observatory will be built above ground. It will have a powerful telescope and camera for making photographs of the earth, the sun, the planets and stars.

Pictures made from the moon will be clearer than any we can make on earth. That's because there is no air around the moon.

Air causes trouble when a camera is aimed through many miles of it. Air carries dust. And it doesn't keep still. Have you noticed how stars seem to twinkle? They really don't. The twinkle comes from the moving air you look through.

It will take many men to run an observatory. There will be scientists, photographers, mechanics, radio engineers, and others.

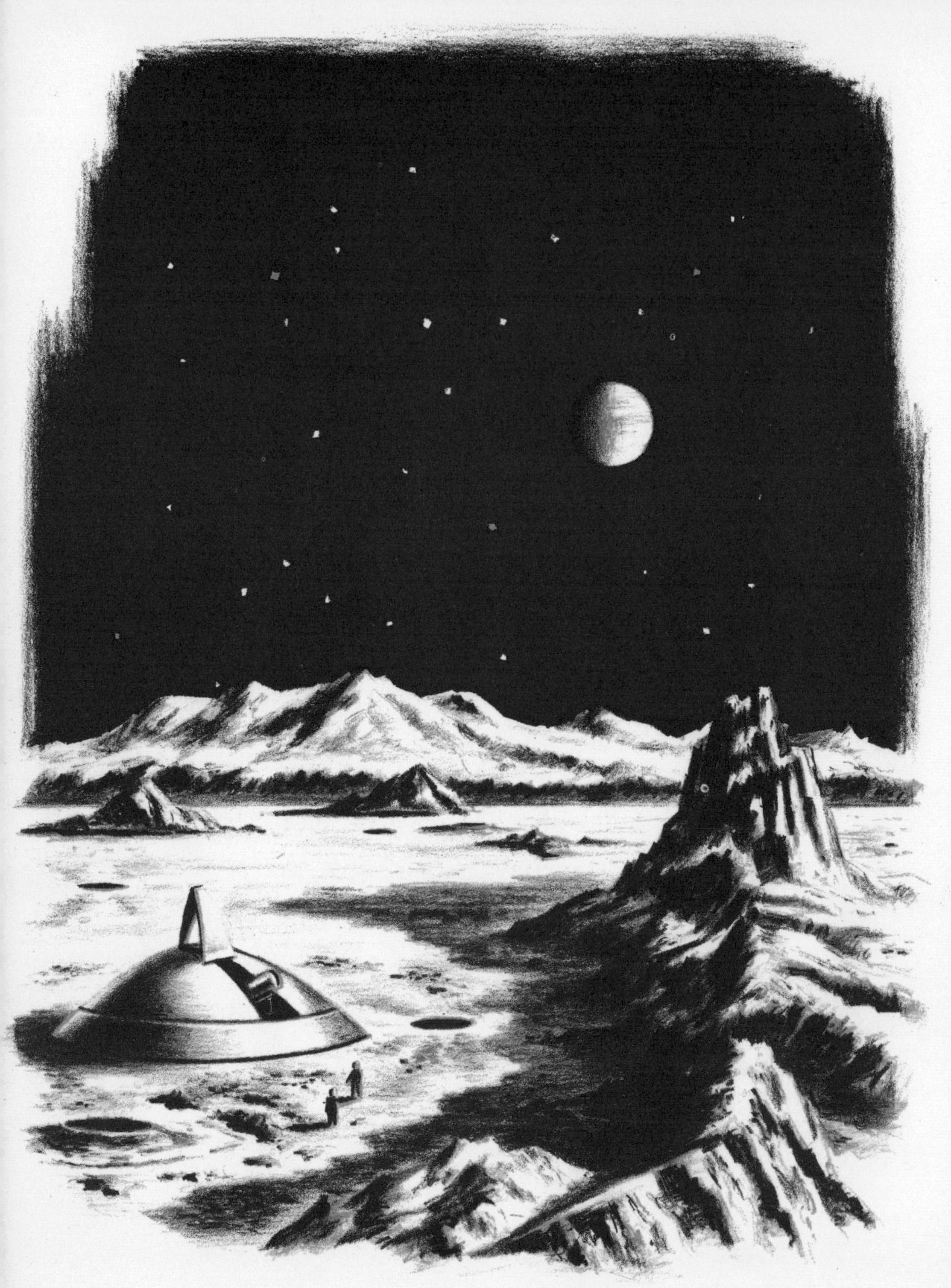

*Astronomers on the moon will photograph the stars.*

These people will need a lot of air. At first the air will be brought from the earth in cylinders. Later the air will be manufactured. How? The rocks on the moon contain oxygen. Scientists know how to get the oxygen by breaking down the rocks with electricity.

Another way to get air is from plants. People and plants get along beautifully. People breathe oxygen and turn it into a gas called carbon dioxide. This is no good for breathing again. But plants take up the carbon dioxide. They eat it up and produce the oxygen that people need.

You may wonder how plants could be grown without sunlight, soil, or rain. This has already been done on earth. Light is supplied by sun lamps. The plants are raised in tanks of water. Crushed rock is added to give the roots something to hold on to. The plants get their food from chemicals which are put into the water.

Gardeners have grown lettuce, tomatoes, cucumbers, cabbage, potatoes, squash, carrots, and other vegetables in tanks of water. Flowers have been raised, too. The moon people can have marigolds on their dinner table.

Plants would grow much taller on the moon. That is because the moon has less gravity than the earth. A man picking tomatoes might need a stepladder.

Wheat and other grains don't do well in tanks. Bread and breakfast cereal would have to come from the earth, along with bacon and hamburgers.

*Fruit and vegetables can be grown in tanks of water.*

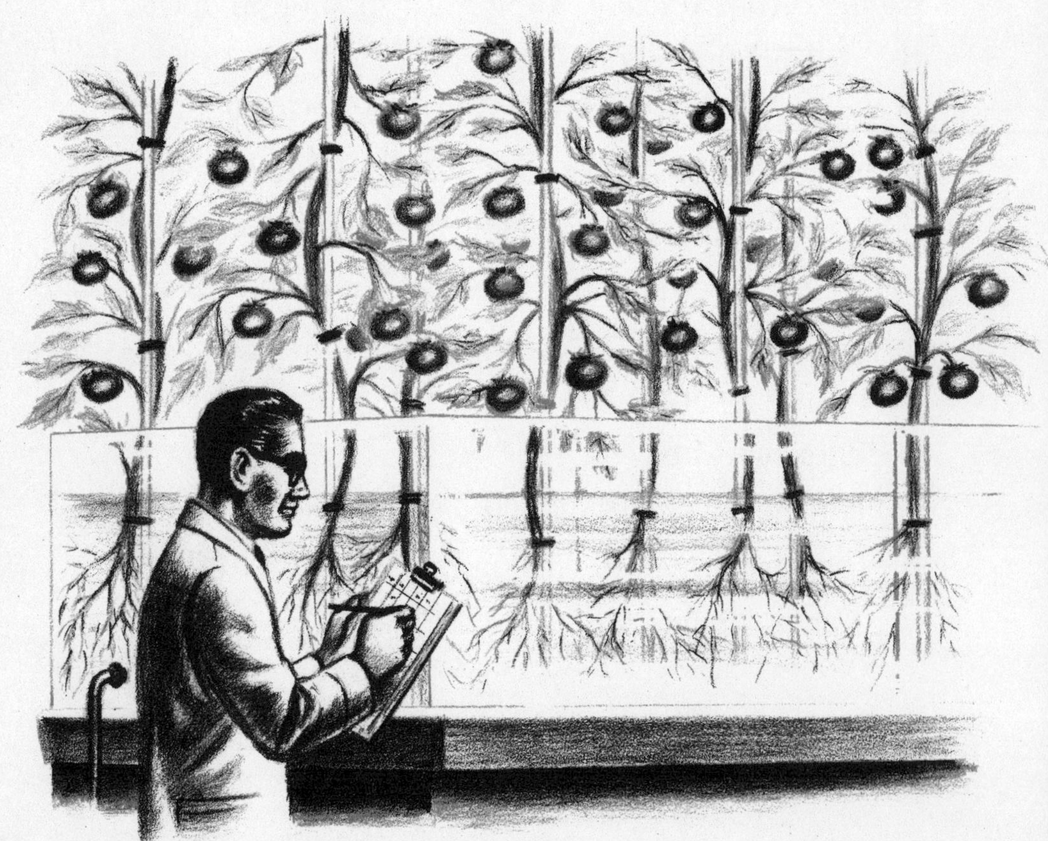

Where would the men on the moon get water? At first it would be brought by rocket ships. But rocks on the moon have hydrogen in them. Water could be manufactured by combining hydrogen and oxygen from rocks.

Electricity would be needed to light the underground rooms, provide heat, run machinery, and do many other jobs. Perhaps an atomic power plant will be built.

Electricity could also be made by using the sun's great heat. Scientists are now working on several plans for doing this.

Construction engineers on the moon will have to get along with few materials. It will be difficult and costly to bring materials from earth.

A great many people will be needed to build the underground chambers and manufacture air and water. Before long there would be a barber shop, a post office, and an Elks Club.

Walking around in a big space suit will be a nuisance. The chances are that moon workers will travel in small tanks run by electric batteries. Each

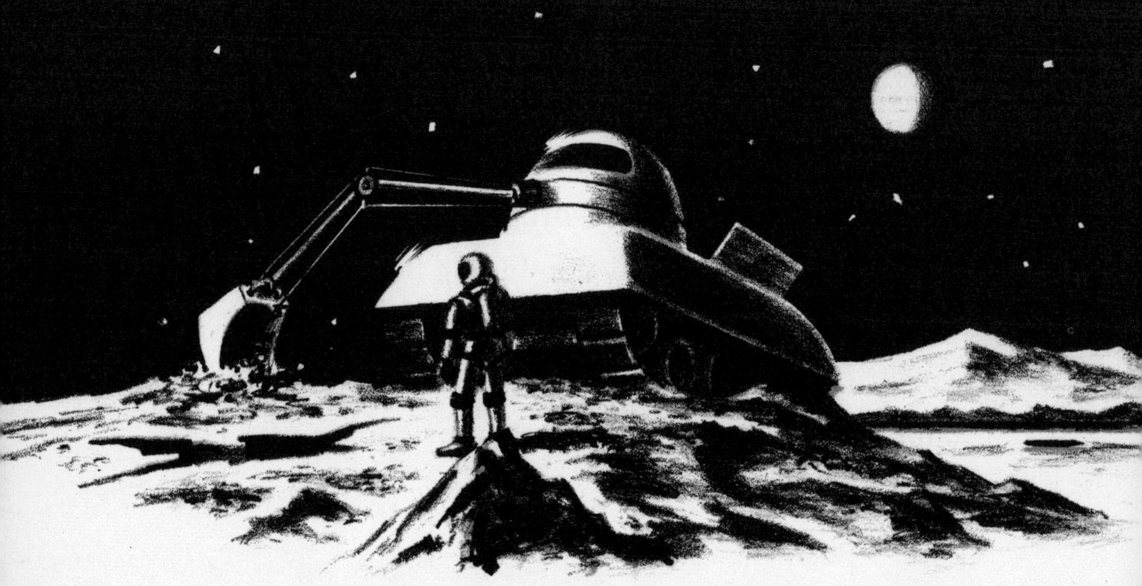

*Steel arms from the tank will scoop up rocks.*

tank would have its own air supply and an air-tight door. The driver would not wear a space suit unless he expected to get out.

Larger tanks could be used for exploring expeditions. The tanks would have steel arms with scoops at the end. Suppose the driver wanted a sample of minerals. He would steer the tank to the spot. The scoop would dig into the ground and come up with a bucketful of rocks and dust. These would be dumped into a bin on the tank. The driver would not step outside of his air-tight compartment.

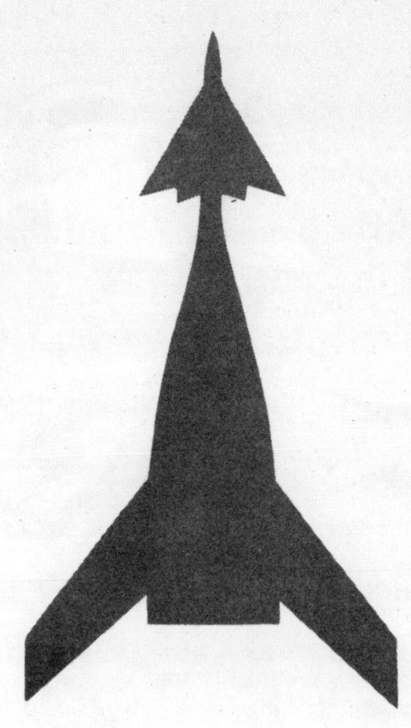

# 11

## WHY DO WE CARE?

The United States and the Soviet Union are spending millions and millions of dollars on rockets. Lives have been lost in building and testing rockets. More lives will be lost before space travel becomes as safe as travel by trains and airplanes.

Why do we care about going to the moon? Is the moon worth all we are spending to get there?

Those are good questions to think about. One of the rocket pioneers, G. Edward Pendray, has some interesting answers.

He says the first reason for going to the moon is man's thirst for adventure. This is what makes you want to explore a stream or take a road you have never tried.

The second reason is our thirst for knowledge. It's the same as your reason for reading this book. You want to know more.

Another reason is man's thirst for wealth. We don't know what we'll find on the moon. But there may be new and valuable kinds of metals and minerals. Someday girls may wear engagement rings with precious gems from the moon.

Finally there is a military reason. The country that controls the moon might have an advantage in war. It might learn things we have no idea of now.

Could a missile be sent from the moon to the

earth? No one knows for sure. But the possibility is frightening.

The moon looks beautiful to us now. We would feel differently if it were loaded with hydrogen bombs that could be aimed at the earth.

Of course that need not happen. Mr. Pendray and other thoughtful people say the moon should be ruled by the United Nations. No one country should control the moon.

If the United Nations had charge of the moon, all countries could use it for scientific experiments.

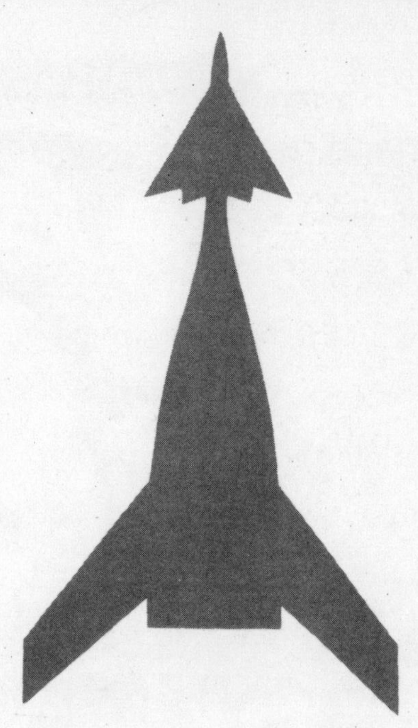

# 12

## NEXT STOP: MARS

Scientists are even more excited about going to Mars than visiting the moon. For years there have been arguments about Mars.

There is good reason to think there are plants on Mars. During the year some areas are green. Later

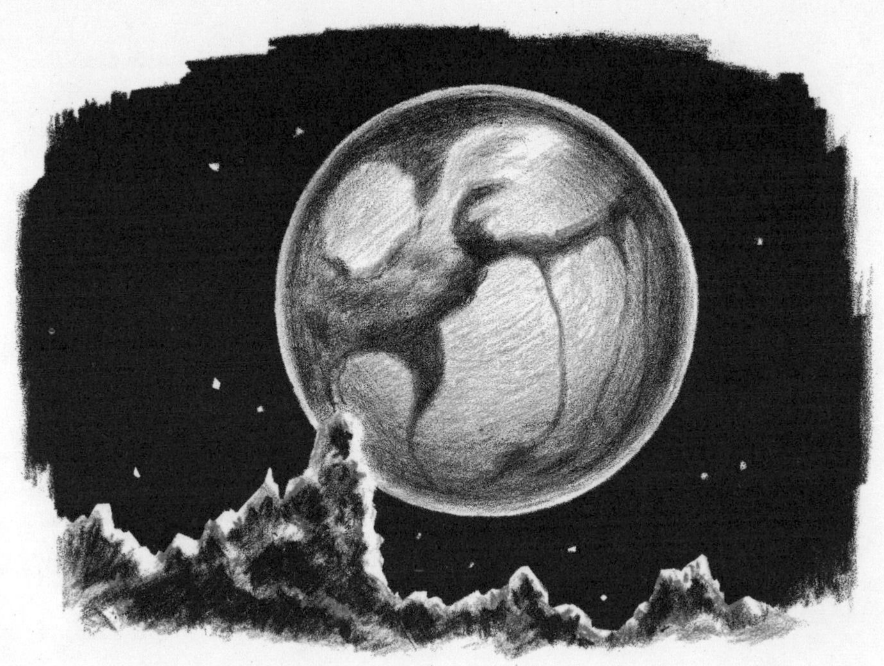

*Mars would look like this from one of its moons.*

they change color, something like the way our fields and woods turn brown in winter.

Mars is a long way from us. Like the earth, it circles the sun. At its closest point Mars is 36,000,000 miles from earth. The sun is 93,000,000 miles from us. The moon is quite close to us—only 240,000 miles.

Some scientists say we'll get to Mars before the

year 2000. Drawings of a space ship to Mars have already been made.

The ship must carry a heavy load of fuel for the long journey. It must carry food and other supplies to last more than two years. The round trip will take that long. A big space ship will be needed to haul the fuel and supplies.

The trip to Mars will begin from a space station in orbit around the earth. The station will always move at a terrific speed. This means the rocket ship will get a flying start.

*To land on Mars a space ship would need wings.*

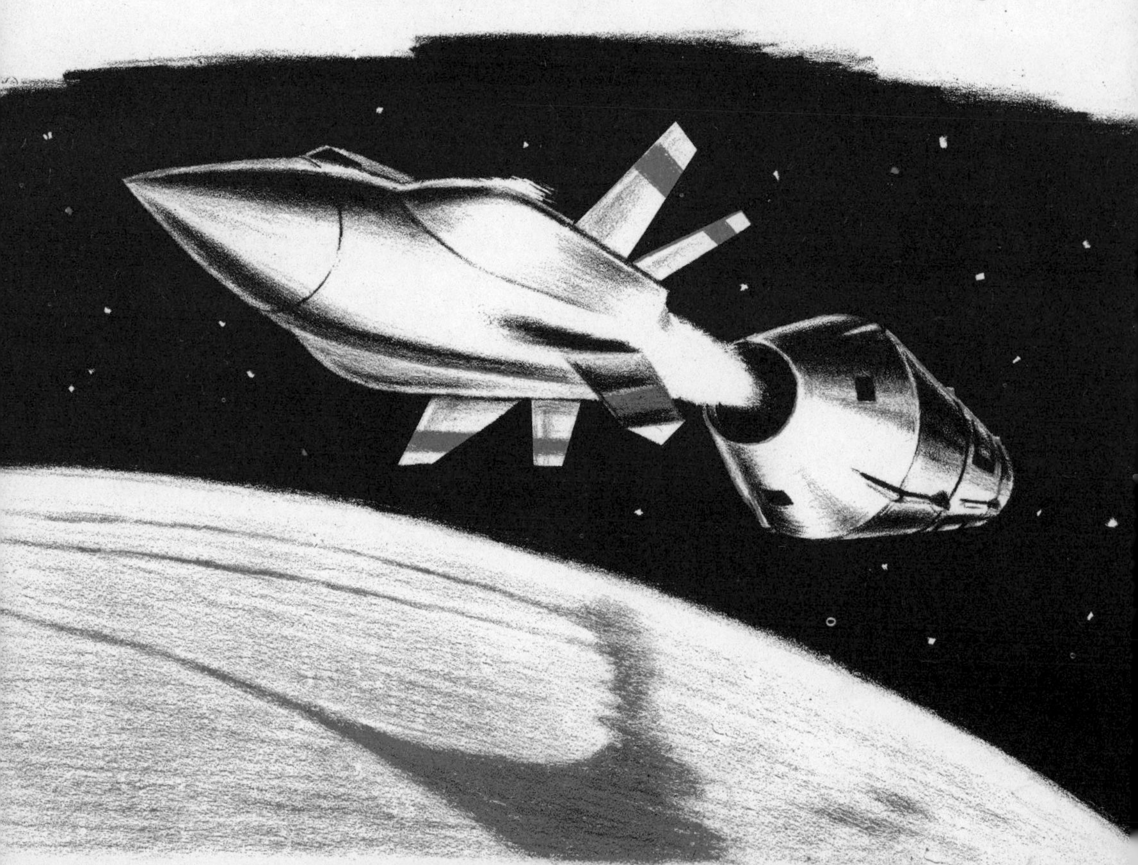

The pilot will fire his motors just enough to gain extra speed and leave the orbit of the space station. Then the ship will coast through space for 260 days. When it gets close to Mars, it won't land. It will circle the planet.

A small rocket ship with wings will be needed to go through the thin blanket of air around Mars. This small ship will be carried by the big space ship.

Explorers in space suits will transfer to the little ship. They will spiral down for a landing on the red planet. The world will be waiting eagerly for news of what the first visitors discover.

A day on Mars is only half an hour longer than a day on earth. Temperatures are cooler there. The summer temperature probably does not go above 86 degrees. At night it falls way below zero.

Mars is believed to be mostly a desert. It has some water but no large lakes or seas. Through a telescope, mysterious lines can be seen on Mars. They look something like a network of irrigation canals. In fact, some astronomers once called them canals. This idea has been given up. But nobody knows what the lines really are.

The first visitors may find the answer.

The explorers will plant a flag. They will collect samples of rocks and soil and plants. They will make tests with various instruments. They will have plenty to talk about as they return to their little rocket ship.

A few hundred miles up they will meet the big space ship that has been circling Mars. They will transfer to it. Then they will start the long journey back to the space station.

The bright planet Venus is closer to the earth than Mars is. You might think it would be explored first.

The trouble with Venus is that no one has ever seen its surface. The planet is always covered with a thick cloud. Beneath that cloud there may be ocean or desert.

When we know more about space travel, we shall try to reach Venus.

# INDEX

## ABOUT THE AUTHORS OF THIS BOOK

ALEXANDER L. CROSBY and NANCY LARRICK, new as a writing team, have been writing separately for many years.

Mr. Crosby, who was born in Maryland and grew up in California, has worked as a carpenter's helper, bridge builder, newspaperman, and book editor. Since 1944 he has been a free-lance writer.

Nancy Larrick, who is Mrs. Crosby in private life, is a native Virginian who migrated to New York. Author of the popular *Parent's Guide to Children's Reading,* she is a past president of the International Reading Association. She has been a teacher and a book editor, and now devotes her time to free-lance writing.

The Crosbys live in Greenwich Village, in New York City.

## ABOUT THE ILLUSTRATOR OF THIS BOOK

DENNY MCMAINS specializes in aviation and space illustration. He has illustrated several books in this area, including *The Story of Aviation* and *Planes That Made History.* For the *Golden Book Encyclopedia,* he provided the illustrations for the sections on rockets, aviation, and space.

Mr. McMains has made aviation his hobby since boyhood, when he constructed model airplanes and studied their technical design. Born in Pennsylvania, he now lives in New York City.

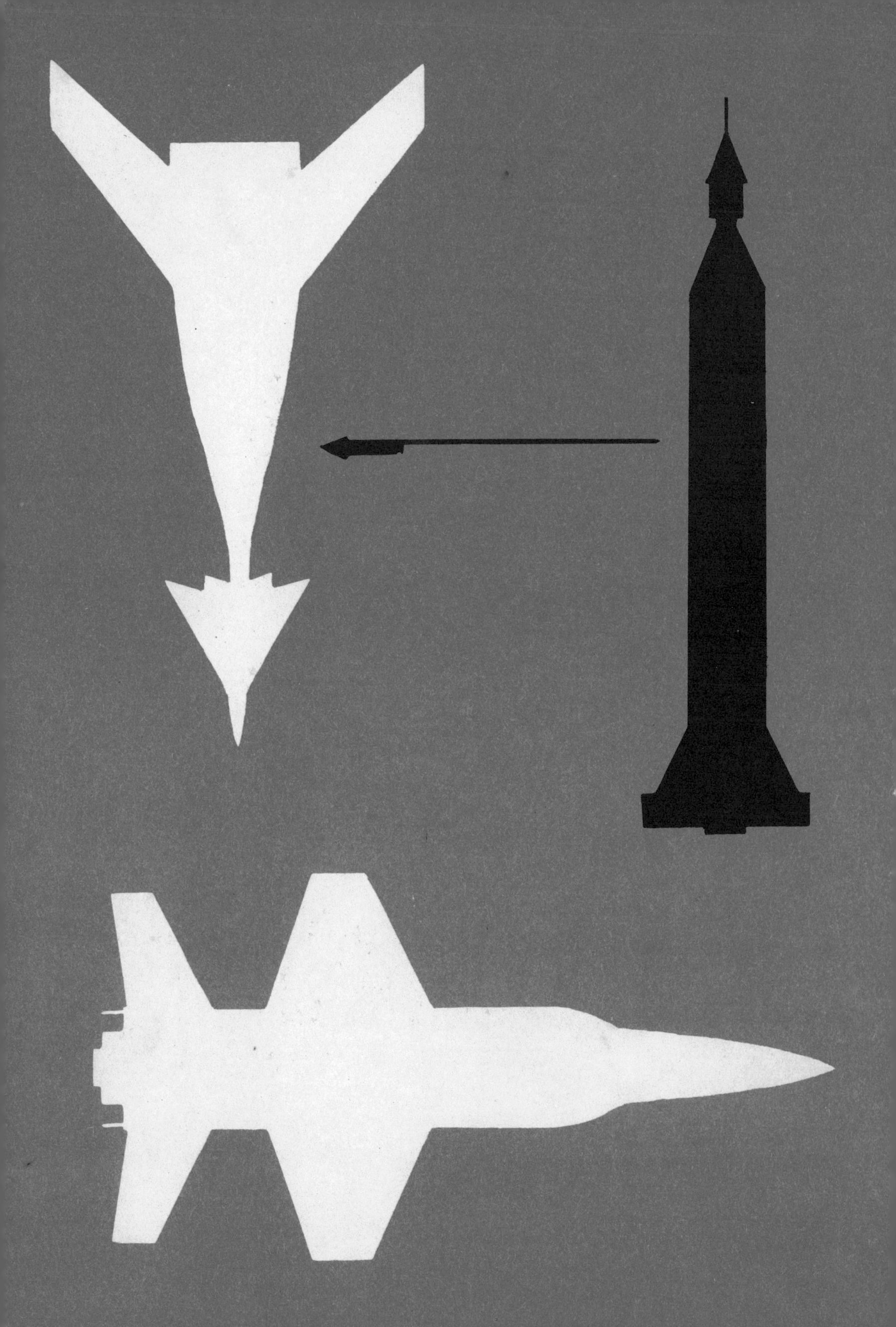